7X METHOD

The Truth About Food & Your Body That's Never Been Told Until Now

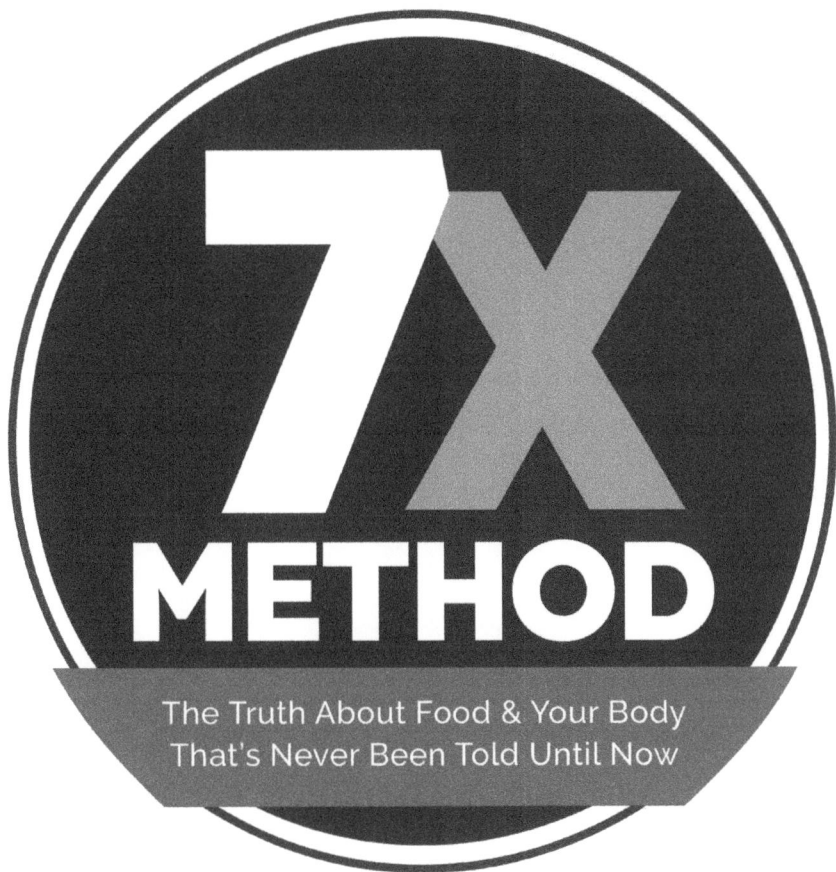

DR. SARAH DOYLE

PT, DPT, CFMP, DACBN

ISBN 978-1-9610938-8-1 (Hardcover Book)

ISBN 979-8-9873816-6-3 (Softcover Book)

ISBN 979-8-9873816-7-0 (eBook)

Published by Silversmith Press–Houston, Texas

www.silversmithpress.com

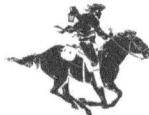

SILVERSMITH
PRESS

Contents

Acknowledgments

Don Doyle: Dad, you always encouraged me to work for myself. Thanks for always being accessible and helping with my business plans and spreadsheets!

Ellen Doyle: Mom, thanks for always having nutritious, home-cooked meals for us every day when we were growing up, for teaching me how to cook at an early age, and then trusting me to cook the family dinners, unsupervised, at age 13!

Katherine Benfante: My younger sister; I couldn't have gotten my doctorate without you helping with my physics equations. It meant a lot to me that you proofread my doctoral thesis and helped edit it, even though your engineering brain does not enjoy medicine like mine does. And thanks for being my guinea pig as I pioneered technology with my app and coaching business. Sometimes I feel like *you're* the big sister!

Sister Stephanie Gillis: Our conversations over the years are priceless; there are few people that I can just geek out to about healthcare and medicine. I appreciate your conventional medical brain as an ARNP vs. my functional medicine brain; we don't always agree, and it's great! You guys are my rocks. I love you all and can't imagine life without you. We truly are a blessed family.

Christine Curran: No woman works as hard as you and I do. I'm so glad we've been able to push each other throughout the years, even though we've gone in completely opposite directions professionally. I look forward to sharing future successes!

Brooks Braun, My Mentor: Amigo, you opened my eyes to the quantic realm, patiently taught me the fundamentals, and charged me with the duty to share this information with the world ...aquí vamos!

Finally, I thank You, **God**, for all Your guidance along my path in life. Countless times per day, I turn to **Jesus** and receive His direction. I am where I am in life because of Him. Amen!

Introduction

It's 6:40 AM on Friday and you're running late. You've been looking forward to a dinner party with your friends whom you haven't seen in ages. Work was crazy this week, the kid's homework was out of control, and you had every intention of trying on clothes a couple of days ago to make sure your outfit was ready to go. However, things aren't going as planned. You have tried on seven outfits so far, and *nothing* in your closet fits. Feeling disgusted and mortified, you say to yourself, "*How did this happen? Working from home in my PJs? Have I been stress eating that much?*"

There are few things in life that sting our pride more than when you have to go out immediately to buy a larger size pair of pants! If that resonates with you today, you're not alone, and you have the right book in your hands. This scenario, or something similar, has happened to millions of people around the world, but now it doesn't have to. In this book, you will learn how you can reduce your bloating, increase your energy, and reset your metabolism in as little as seven days. The 7X Method will work for you even when *all other* diets and programs have failed. In fact, nothing like this has been pushed mainstream, even though it's been practiced in remote regions of the world for decades. Yes, this method of eating has been used to reverse disease, restore youth, and lose weight for more than 50 years.

Do you sometimes feel like your body has betrayed you? Autoimmune diseases and food allergies have skyrocketed in the past decade. So has the amount of conflicting and confusing information available to us on the internet. If you have ever experienced–or are currently experiencing–chronic indigestion, painful bloating, embarrassing gas, toxic constipation, unpredictable diarrhea, unsightly rashes, or pathological blood sugar dysregulation issues, you especially need this information. The secret is learning to fuel your body based on what it needs according to your own natural biorhythms. Don't worry about what that means just yet, it will all make sense soon. Just take in the idea that you give your body *what* it needs *when* it needs it.

Essentially, we are using specific foods ingested at specific times to communicate to the body how to make very drastic changes. There are thousands upon thousands of processes happening as we make this transition. Please keep focused on your outcome and create positive visualizations on how you see your "new self" fitting into your "skinny jeans," feeling confident in your swimsuit, and being the envy of your peers. The 7X Method isn't just about physical changes, it's about mental and spiritual growth as well.

Getting rid of the leaky gut and brain will be one of the first noticeable milestones. Enjoy your increased energy levels and clarity of thought. In time, you will advance into a deeper understanding of things in general. It's hard to explain, but I feel like a light bulb went on in my head. You will just have to learn from personal experience how transformative this really is.

You see, once you start eating like this consistently, you will experience positive shifts in other facets of your life. You may notice improved or more fulfilling relationships. Maybe your career will advance, or you will finally go out on your own like you have dreamed about for years. Something in the brain just clicks. Personally, I began to live with more purpose in everything that I do. Everything is done with intention. I noticed myself feeling more at ease and abundant. One year from now, you are going to reflect on this day and be so amazed by yourself and your metamorphosis.

Best of all, there's no counting macros or calories, which modern science now proves was the wrong approach all along! Yes, that's right. No wonder so many people think they are doing all the "right" things and keep getting the "wrong" results. It's not your fault! The 7X Method will teach you how to choose foods according to the quantum of energy it has, at the time of day your body needs it, which means you will use that energy and not store it as fat and inflammation.

Don't worry, it's way easier than it might sound, and this book will explain everything. For now, just take a deep breath and get ready to "unlearn" some things that have kept you stuck in a cycle of frustration about your health and weight. I've heard it said that the definition of insanity is to *keep doing the same thing over and over, expecting different results*. You need to do something different to get something different and believe me, the 7X Method makes the difference! Not only will this approach change your relationship with food, but when your body systems are energized and optimized, and when you are feeling revitalized with a strong sense of well-being, it will totally change your life! If you are tired of low energy, acid reflux, metabolic issues, hormone issues, low libido, and just feeling poorly, if you've been struggling to feel "like you" and have your vitality back, welcome to the moment that can change everything!

The first myth I want to dispel is the idea in the diet industry that there's no one-size-fits-all eating plan. WRONG! Everybody needs the sun, everybody needs water, and everybody needs specific types of energy at specific times of the day to nourish the specific systems of the body that we all have. While the 7X Method is customizable for preferences, the guidelines provided work for all body types.

For example, maybe you're the husband whose wife just gave birth, but *you* look like the one pregnant! Or maybe you're the busy mom whose second child is finally at the stage where you can actually take a break and think about yourself, and you realize you haven't had sex with your husband in *months!* Not because you don't love him, but because you aren't feeling very sexy yourself, even if you did have the energy for it . . . which you don't. Many women experience hormonal imbalances for years after giving birth, including but not limited to decreased progesterone, decreased thyroid, increased or decreased estrogen, and altered cortisol levels. The effects of stress and late-night feedings negatively affect our internal clock by exacerbating hormonal imbalances. The 7X Method of eating will nourish your endocrine system and support the re-balancing of your hormone levels, so you can feel like yourself again–energetic and full of desire (especially early to mid-afternoon and into the evening!).

Now, this might sound like a tall order, and you might be wondering how I can say all of these things. Let me tell you, I didn't make this up, this is not theory. I mentioned previously that this eating method has been implemented in other parts of the world as a healing diet for over half a century! Let me tell you how I came to learn about it.

For the past 20 years, I took high doses of digestive enzymes with every meal because I would get heartburn at night and stomach cramps during the day. I had terrible digestion. I started eating and living the 7X Method in August 2020. Within a couple of weeks, the heartburn and poor digestive symptoms were gone. I haven't needed a digestive enzyme since implementing this diet. Many of my food sensitivities went away as well. I used to have diarrhea whenever I ate fruit, but now I eat fruit every morning.

It all started because I was on a quest for answers to my own digestive and health issues. In my travels, I met a healer in Central America who explained this way of eating that brought health and vitality to his people. It wasn't like anything I had heard before, but it made sense on a scientific level, so I decided to give it a try. When I implemented the program, it made a night-and-day difference almost immediately. Because of my background in natural health, I was able to make a few small tweaks to adapt it to be effective for the Western culture and food supply. After eating this way for over a year with my modifications, I have experienced increased energy, decreased bloating, improved digestion, and a clearer mental state–which is what most of America is after too! That's why I'm so excited to bring this revolutionary plan to the mainstream through this book, my coaching program, and other resources. When you get your health back, you get your life back!

Read this book. Change your life. You deserve it. You deserve to have dinner with your friends and hear them say, "Wow, you look amazing, what have you been doing?" You deserve to feel passion in bed with your partner. You deserve to love your body again. Embracing the 7X Method will take you there.

The Calorie is Dead

"Is there a weeklong detox I can do to kickstart my progress and help me not feel so bloated and...blah?" Trendy calorie restriction diets like Prolon, where the client consumes just 770-1,100 calories per day, have made people think that somehow a quick fix will give that permanent slimmer waistline. Nope! Sorry!

As a natural health practitioner and wellness coach, this is one of the most often asked questions by my clients. And while I would love to be the keeper of the magic "quick fix," we have to be realistic. First of all, there's no way to "detox" a lifetime of poor habits, processed foods, and overindulging in junk in just one week. It's just impossible. Permanent results require a permanent shift in behavior. However, that doesn't mean you can't make quick progress in the right direction which will empower you and fuel your determination to make lasting changes that will yield lasting results.

But what if I told you, "You *can* eat the foods that you like (barring processed, conventional, and GMOs), in the amounts that satisfy you, but you just have to change *when* you eat them." Seems too good to be true? It's not. But before I ask you to learn something new, I will first ask you to unlearn the old. You see, for the last 100 years, instead of teaching us how to eat, the diet industry has taught us math. Count calories,[1] count fat grams, eat sugar-free, eat fat-free, measure this, measure that. We've all been doing the math but it's not adding up! It's left us feeling deprived, defeated, and fatter than ever. Let's explore why.

For starters, let's look at the calorie. (Nerd Alert: we are about to get into some "heavy" science, but you will benefit greatly from understanding this information. Stick with me. It will all come together and make sense, even if you aren't a "science" person!)

The definition of a "calorie" according to the Oxford English Dictionary is "the energy needed to raise the temperature of 1 kilogram of water 1 degree celsius." This also referred to as a kilo calorie. We are very familiar with using the calorie as a unit to measure the energy content of food. How is this determined? Scientists use a device called a calorimeter, which is basically a small steel drum container surrounded by water. The food to be analyzed is placed into the steel drum and heated until it is literally burned to ashes. As the temperature rises to heat the food, the temperature of the water also rises. The scientists record the rise in water temperature and correlate that number with how much energy is needed to turn the food to ashes. Essentially, that's how they determine how many calories a certain food has. [2]

Research from McGill University tells us this methodology is flawed and, frankly, I agree. I'm not sure why we use this model. Last time I checked, the human body didn't boil water or create ash. However, we excrete waste via urine, feces, and breath, but certainly not by making ashes.

The caloric model merely estimates how much energy is in a particular food, but it assumes all foods to have the same *type* of energy and impact on the body. Think about it. Don't you feel lighter when you eat fruits and vegetables than when you eat a greasy burger and fries? Even if it's the same number of "calories"? That's because different foods have different energetic properties that our bodies utilize differently.

In our current food model, foods are assigned an energetic value based on the number of grams of macronutrients and the calories they contain, for example, an average apple has about 100 calories, 25 grams of carbohydrates, and a trace amount of protein.[3] One type of diet might restrict a person to 1,200-1,500 calories per day in the short term to achieve the desired weight. Another type of diet would restrict the number of macronutrients you can eat each day. We know of three macronutrients: carbohydrates (4 calories per gram), fats (9 calories per gram), and proteins (4 calories per gram). This model acknowledges that foods should be categorized by their chemical properties. Nowadays, anyone can take an online quiz that will tell you to eat XX grams of protein, YY grams of fat, and ZZ grams of carbs. But at the end of the day, these macros are still counted...we're back to math again.

So, how does the 7X Method, based on quantum energy, compare to our current caloric food model? The 7X Method considers the fact that different types of food have different types of quantum energy. Don't be intimidated by the word *quantum*. The Oxford English Dictionary defines quantum as, "the discrete quantity of energy proportional to the frequency of the radiation that it represents." Keywords: *discrete and quantity*. The definition of "discrete" in mathematics is "objects or data that can be organized into sets according to their characteristics, such as colors or sizes." Make a mental note: *quantum energy can be organized into sets by color or size*. Very important! So, one way of organizing things is by grouping them according to similar characteristics such as grouping lemons, limes, grapefruits, and tangerines together because they belong to the citrus fruit family. Or, grouping golden retrievers, spaniels, pit bulls, and pugs together because they belong to the canine species. These are examples of the discrete data model.

The opposite in mathematics is referred to as "continuous" data, which is data that can take a sequential numerical value, such as weight, height, temperature, calories, etc.[4] When I was 15, I weighed 124 pounds, now that I am 42, I weigh 133 pounds. The bigger I get, the more pounds I weigh. The longer I exist on this planet, the higher my age. The bigger the muffin, the more calories it has. This is the continuous data model.

Do you see where I am going with this? We have been measuring the energetic quality of food using the continuous data model. This is *all wrong*. The energy we get from food should be measured using the discrete data model, by grouping foods into sets based on their respective quantum energetic effect on the body. Don't worry if that's not clicking just yet–it will!

THE WAY IT SHOULD BE

To give you a broad overview, the 7X Method is centered around giving the organs and systems in your body certain types of energy that it requires at certain times of the day. In the 7X Method, we never focus on total calories or macronutrients. This may be the hardest thing to wrap your brain around. But just because we don't count calories, doesn't mean you can eat huge portions of food and still lose weight. Too much energy taken in and not used eventually becomes too much stored energy (fat).

Eating the wrong types of energy at the wrong time of day, like white foods for breakfast, will also cause inflammation, indigestion, and bloating. You see, your body is designed to eat different foods at different times during the day, and learning this secret is powerful because it will unlock your body's ability to create transformation. Your whole life, you have been conditioned to count calories instead of learning about how to fuel your body properly. Fueling your body is more than just knowing "how much," it's about knowing "when" and "what" too. And when you understand the "why," it becomes natural to eat this way. The 7X Method isn't a diet . . . it's a paradigm shift!

As I said before, food is meant to be categorized by its quantum, or *the type of energy* that it possesses. Here's why. All food gets its energy from sunlight (radiation), whether it be directly, as in the case of plants, or indirectly as in the case of animals–because most animals eat plants–and therefore, we indirectly get the sun's energy when we eat that animal. The 7X Method teaches you to follow a natural order which is explained by planetary influences on the body's biological systems, known as your biorhythms. This includes your electrical balance and metabolic function, resulting from the photon energy effects taking place in the body at the microscopic level.

Okay, are your eyes glossing over? Hang in there! Simply put, the energetic effects of the earth's rotation around the sun play a role in the natural rhythms found in both *your body* and *the food you eat*. The key is syncing food's energy with your body's rhythms for optimal health and wellness. This means changing your relationship with food altogether and reprogramming your brain to associate specific foods with specific times of the day. Don't worry, I will tell you exactly what to eat and when to eat it in the coming chapters. Just take in the idea that the timing of when you eat certain foods correlates to the specific needs of your organs and systems within your body. Many people understand that the body regenerates different organs and systems at different times of the day. This means fueling those systems to maintain homeostasis, giving you optimal energy! *This* is how you fight aging from the inside out.

CHAPTER 2

Eating in Rhythm

Sunrise, sunset. Our world is regulated by seasons and rhythms. You may be familiar with circadian rhythm, which is the inherent cycle of approximately 24 hours that influences various biological processes, such as sleep, wakefulness, and digestive activity.[5] We understand that we should sleep at night when it's dark and be awake during the day when it's light. Our bodies give us clues by the way we feel, that this is a good idea. If you try to stay up all night, how do you feel the next day? Not great. Eventually, your body begins to break down if you don't give it rest at the proper time. But what about eating at the appropriate time? More importantly, eating the right foods at the correct time? How do you feel when you eat late at night? Not great, I would imagine. We aren't meant to eat in the middle of the night. Our bodies perform better when fueled at the right times of the day. Our bodies also perform better when fueled with the right type of energy–food–at the right times of the day.

Here in this quantum realm, we find photon energy as the primary stimulus for the human body. The physics formula is E=hf, where E=energy, h=Planck's constant (just a number like pi, 3.14), and f=frequency.[6] A photon is a particle of light that contains electromagnetic radiation, has no mass and travels at the speed of light at different frequencies. A frequency means how many times a wave peaks and troughs in a specific period of time. This concept is like speed when you drive your car at 65 miles (104 km) per hour. You know that the more times per minute the wheel goes around, the higher your speed. Similarly, the laws of physics state that light's energy is proportional to its frequency. So, the higher the frequency, the greater the energy.

I like the following diagram below because it shows different kinds of energetic frequencies and compares them to objects that we are familiar with. For example, you can see that the human body radiates heat at a higher frequency than a microwave but at a lower frequency than infrared or visible light.

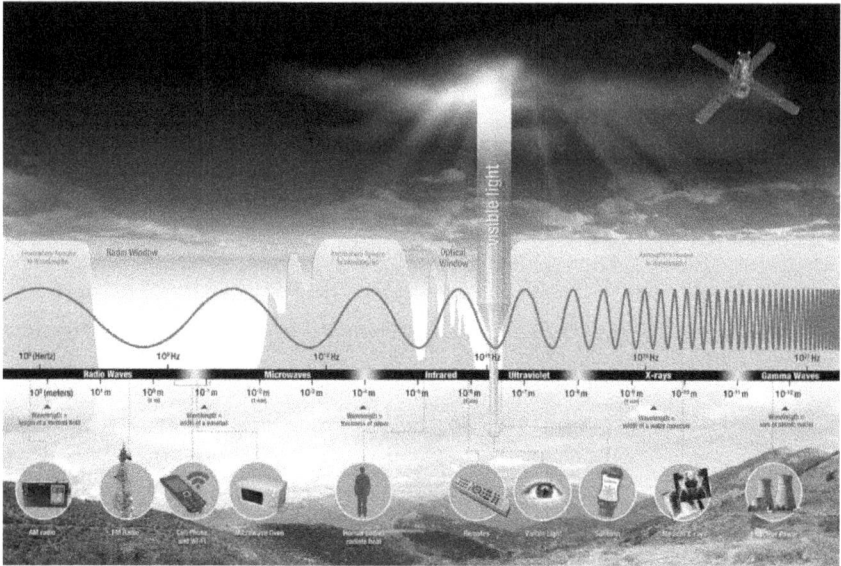

PC: https://ftloscience.com/wavelength-frequency-energy/

Let's explore more about how light and circadian rhythm impact your body. It starts at sunrise when your eyes see the first light of the day. The light emitted from the sun is what we call white light, which is a combination of all colors of light in the visible spectrum, what we learned as children to be all the colors of the rainbow. Contained within that is blue light, and its specific frequency activates the melanopsin cells in the eye's retina. Then the signal travels along the optic nerves and communicates directly with the suprachiasmatic nucleus (SCN) in the brain, a small area of the hypothalamus above the optic chiasm.[7] More on the SCN in a moment. Don't let the big "science-y" words trip you up. Basically, the light signals the brain to get up and get going! When light hits your eyes, it also suppresses the production of melatonin which is the hormone that makes you sleep.

Now, let's go back to the suprachiasmatic nucleus (SCN); this little guy has a very important role, and you've probably never even heard of it. To break it down, supra means "above." Chiasmatic refers to the optic chiasm, the part of the brain where the nerves from each eye connect and crisscross. Nucleus means it's a like a hub or control center. Okay, so our brain has a control center that responds to light, and it is located where our optic nerves from our eyes meet up. The SCN is the centralized pacemaker of circadian timing and regulates most circadian rhythms in the body.[8] So, think of the SCN as your body's internal clock.

It's been discovered in recent years that our organs and systems each have individual circadian rhythms, which means our organs take turns working and resting. Stop and think about that for a moment. At the basic level, we are a collection of cells and systems. Our cells go through a process of cellular regeneration, which means each organ and body system, i.e., cardiovascular system, lymphatic system, nervous system, etc. also go through a process of regeneration. So, the SCN is the control center for all the different circadian rhythms of your organs and systems. Think of it like the air traffic control system at an airport. Someone has to regulate activity and tell the planes when to take off and land because if all the planes start down the runway at the same time, you'll have a mess on your hands.

So, your master body clock, the SCN, is stimulated by light energy and it sets the pace for all the other circadian rhythms of the organs and systems of your body, or what we might call, peripheral clocks. Many hormones involved in metabolism, such as insulin,[9] glucagon,[10] adiponectin,[11] corticosterone,[12] leptin, and ghrelin,[13,14] have shown circadian patterns. This may be because the central clock (SCN) regulates metabolism and energy homeostasis in tissues outside of the brain[15] by controlling the activity of certain metabolic enzymes and systems which are[16] involved in: cholesterol metabolism, amino acid regulation, drug and toxin metabolism, the citric acid cycle (which is how we get ATP, the currency of energy), and glycogen and glucose metabolism. By now it should be obvious to you why it is important to get to bed by 10 p.m.

FIRST THING'S FIRST

Now, before you work on anything else in your health, the most important thing is to regulate and manage the way you stimulate your SCN, your master clock, and the circadian rhythm of your sleep-wake cycle. You need sleep to be healthy and to lose weight!

It's common for people to stay up watching television past midnight or stay on smart devices which emit those blue rays we talked about earlier. When you do this, you are signaling your SCN that it's wake-up time, and you are suppressing your melatonin production. No wonder so many people have sleep issues! Then they wake up for work feeling sleep-deprived and use stimulants like coffee and energy drinks to cope with fatigue and drowsiness. It's like you can't get your plane off the ground!

Not only that, but internally, all the other rhythms of the body are being disrupted as a result. This circadian rhythm disruption is an all too prevalent feature of modern-day society, associated with an increase in pro-inflammatory diseases[17] such as obesity, diabetes, autoimmune diseases, cancers, and heart disease. Symptoms vary but can include atherosclerosis (plaque build-up on arteries), gastrointestinal inflammation, rashes, depression (brain inflammation), fatigue, heartburn, asthma, blood sugar dysregulation, and more. These are further exacerbated by stress which causes your adrenal glands to become overworked. Your adrenal glands produce hormones that help you regulate blood pressure, immune system, metabolism, your body's response to stress, and other important functions. And guess what? The circadian rhythm of your adrenal glands has them in a state of rest and restoration between 10 p.m. and 2 a.m. every night. What do you think you should be doing at that time in order to let your adrenal glands rest so they can prepare to manage the stress of tomorrow? That's right, sleep. If you go to bed after midnight, your adrenals have already lost half their time to repair themselves. So, the next day, when it's time to fire up your adrenal glands, what do you think will happen? Well, it will be like putting a broken airplane on the runway. Not good.

Many of the inflammatory symptoms people suffer from can be reversed with proper food and behavioral modifications, which we will get into in the coming chapters. The 7X Method is a way of eating and living to help you reduce cellular inflammation, eliminate the physical stress of cellular residue from poor digestion, and maximize cellular and electrical systems within the body. In other words, it will make you feel great! But step one is getting the circadian rhythm of your sleep-wake cycle straightened out because this is the most critical clock in your body. Here's how. . .

STEP 1: SET A REGULAR SLEEP SCHEDULE

You probably already knew this was important, but maybe you didn't understand why. Ideally, you should be going to bed by 10:00 p.m. so that you are waking up naturally around 6 a.m., even on the weekends. I touched on this earlier but there's a lot going on when you wake up, open your eyes, and look out the window. First, the sunlight hits the ganglion cells in the retina, travels down the optic nerves, and signals the SCN. *Good morning, brain!* The SCN then delivers another signal using a relaxing brain chemical, the neurotransmitter called GABA (gamma-aminobutyric acid), which stops the activity of the sympathetic nervous system (your fight-or-flight response). Finally, melatonin production is discontinued for the rest of the day.[18] Let that really sink in: viewing blue light stops the release of melatonin, your sleep hormone. Ever wonder why you feel sluggish waking up on a rainy day? It's because you don't have a sufficient light signal to jump-start this process!

STEP 2: SLEEP IN DARKNESS

There's as much happening in your body when the sun goes down. As night approaches, a decrease in light signals the mela-nopsin cells in the eye's retina to inhibit the activity of the SCN. In other words, it's time to land the plane. This ultimately activates the sympathetic (fight-or-flight) nervous system to stimulate the pineal gland to release melatonin into circulation to prepare your body for sleep.[19] Isn't it so cool how our bodies work in predictive cycles like this? Unless, of course, you are using artificial light in the evenings. This is where blue-light-blocking glasses can be helpful. Ideally, you should have nothing but water after 7 p.m. so that your pancreas can stop releasing insulin to regulate blood sugar, and your pineal gland can release melatonin at 9 p.m. Make this your goal.

Many of us stay up two or more hours later on weekends than we do during the work week. This is called social jet lag, and it negatively affects the circadian rhythm of all our systems.[20] Being a shift worker, having jet lag from traveling across time zones, as well as social jet lag, have been shown to have detrimental effects on health.[21]

On a side note, the frequency of orange light is not picked up on the melanopsin cells but is picked up on the rods and cones, permitting you to see.[22] This is one reason why an orange Hima-layan salt lamp makes a safe nightlight for trips to the bathroom;

it allows you to navigate safely but won't disrupt your circadian rhythm.

CIRCADIAN RHYTHMS OF DISEASE

As mentioned earlier, our organs, for the most part, have their own circadian clocks.[23,24] It's logical to think that it's impossible for an organ or system to function at full throttle 24/7; it needs time to rest and repair. It also implies that these organs and systems have energetic needs at specific times of the day to restore their vitality and continue to function at optimal levels. These electrical needs are provided by the food we eat. Each type of food has a specific type of energy too, and when we match the food with the type of energy we need at the time of day that we need it, we can achieve optimal wellness in our bodies. This factor has never been addressed until now and it is the missing link as to why and how all other diets and eating systems don't work, why they cannot sustain weight loss, and why most of us fail. Sure, crash diets work at first, but eventually, side effects come to the surface.

You may have tried them all...Atkins, Keto, Vegan, Paleo, ProLon, Carnivore, FODMAP, Plant-Based; the list is endless. More often than not, previous eating patterns are eventually resumed. These fad diets are challenging to stick to at the very least and can sometimes be dangerous at worst. I recall when my mom fainted in a restaurant and consequently was hospitalized for kidney damage that was later attributed to long-term adherence to the carb-restricted diet. The low-carb, high-fat diet also caused me to have elevated triglycerides, and I still can't look at bacon! There are many diets to choose from, but you have to ask yourself, "Is this something I can do for the rest of my life?" The 7X Method is designed to be something *you can follow for the rest of your life*. Regardless of whether or not your goal is to lose weight, it will benefit you to understand how to eat for your body's circadian rhythms to maintain general health and avoid chronic disease.

As mentioned before, circadian rhythm disruption is involved in the onset of pro-inflammatory diseases, but we are just beginning to learn how diseases also follow circadian rhythms. As mentioned earlier, almost every cell has an inherent circadian clock mechanism that keeps time and has clock output genes specific to its tissue.[25] Circadian rhythm clock genes play a significant role in the development of cancer, loss of cognition, and neurodegenerative disease, like dementia.[26] The occurrence of sudden cardiac death from heart attacks also follows a strong diurnal rhythm, with the highest number occurring around the early morning hours during the transition from sleep to wake.[27]

Research shows that a high-fat diet, like the typical fast-food American diet, stimulates a massive reorganization of specific metabolic pathways, leading to general remodeling of the liver clock. It is precisely the nutritional challenge of eating garbage, and not the actual development of obesity, that causes the reprogramming of the liver's circadian clock. Luckily, the effects of a poor diet on the liver clock are reversible.[28]

NAFLD (non-alcoholic fatty liver disease) is the most common liver disease in developed countries. It is characterized by the accumulation of triglycerides in the liver cells without excess alcohol intake.[29] Most people don't realize that it is entirely reversible. The root cause of NAFLD is often high-stress levels combined with poor diet choices, diets high in sugar, and seed oils like fried foods, fast foods, etc. The disease pathology shares several characteristics of metabolic syndrome, such as type 2 diabetes mellitus, insulin resistance, abdominal obesity, arterial hypertension, and dyslipidemia.

Circadian rhythms of cholesterol, lipid, and glucose metabolism are also closely related to this disease's metabolic dysfunctions. Meaning that synchronizing circadian rhythms can help move the liver disease in a positive direction.[30] Lifestyle modification as primary therapy for the management of NAFLD is strongly supported by clinical evidence.[31]

The moon has daily, weekly, monthly, and annual cycles that affect our physiology. For example, the Royal Melbourne Hospital in Australia analyzed over 4,000 stroke patients between 2004-2011. They found that most strokes occurred during spring or summer, during the first quarter or full moon, and were least likely to occur between the hours of 12:00 a.m. and 6:00 a.m.[32]

Although the cause of depression is multifactorial, circadian rhythm disruption may play a role in the onset of a depressive episode. For example, I used to get depressed every winter when

I lived up North, and I self-medicated by going to the tanning bed a few times per week. It is commonly known that during the winter months, when days are shorter and nights are longer, certain people are predisposed to seasonal affective disorder (SAD), where they experience depressive symptoms during winter that resolve in spring.

We need sunlight to synthesize vitamin D in the skin. Unfortunately, many people have low vitamin D levels despite taking supplemental vitamin D. I think the public became aware of this during the COVID-19 pandemic. God designed us to be outside in nature, absorbing the sun's energy.

Light, Energy, and the Food We Eat

We all have our own unique health attributes and challenges inherited from our parents, such as heart disease or diabetes. The genetics of which can either lie dormant or be triggered to be turned on by external environmental influences, gut dysbiosis (poor digestion), and different types of stressors.[33] You are special and unique in this world. However, we have one thing in common: We all live on this planet, which has a direct magnetic and energetic relationship with the sun. At first, this may seem trivial and esoteric, but if you think about it, all life on this planet results from this predictable and precisely timed planetary relationship. Stay with me.

This is because our internal clock (SCN), which rules all cellular metabolism, results from these changing energetic fields. It is this electric "charge" that our endocrine system uses to communicate "what" and "when" to start or stop a metabolic function. For example, insulin, the thyroid, and even the microbiota in your gut follow a circadian rhythm.[34] These metabolic processes are easily decoupled from the light-driven SCN when food intake falls out of sync with normal daily patterns of activity.[35]

Here's the take-home message: The circadian rhythms of our organs and systems are affected by sunlight. This light energy also has electromagnetic radiation. Different foods possess different kinds of energetic qualities. You already knew these things before you picked up this book; it's just that nobody ever explained the relationship among these concepts before now.

You know that darkness is the absence of light, black is the absence of color, and white light can be separated into colors by refracting light with a prism. What makes each color different is the specific energetic frequency of that color of light. A rainbow is a phenomenon in which white light is separated into its individual parts based on its energetic wavelength or frequency. When you look at a rainbow, you can recognize that each color you see results from a specific frequency for that color. The following diagram can help you visualize this. The electric charge or frequency of a particular food is represented by its color much of the time as well.

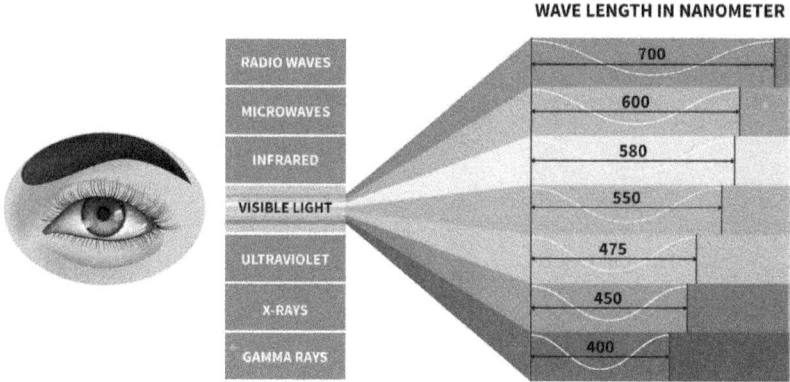

WAVE LENGTH IN NANOMETER

PC: Burlington County Eye Physicians

This is why foods are categorized into seven different food groups in the 7X Method. Because our organs and systems function based on their retrospective circadian rhythms or local clock rhythms. They have specific nutritional needs at certain times of the day. Therefore, they respond to different frequencies of energy in foods.

The burning question that I often get when I tell people I learned this from a group of natives while traveling is: "How did they know which foods, times, organs, and systems go together?"

The body works magnetically through the ionization of every-thing, including food.[36] Elements are pulled apart, destructed, and reconstructed. You drink water (H_2O) and exhale carbon dioxide (CO_2). You eat chicken and rice with veggies at dinner, and the following morning, you hopefully have a bowel movement. It doesn't look like what was on your plate last night because your body reconstructed it molecule by molecule. This we know. But how did they know that the dominant energy received from the sun at 1 p.m. is like the energy of chicken and steak? They measured it with a spectrophotometer. A spectro-what? According to a US government agency called the National Institute of Standards and Technology, "Spectrophotometry is a quantitative measurement technique that allows scientists to investigate the optical properties of materials over a wide wavelength range, from the ultraviolet to the visible and infrared spectral regions. It involves measuring the ratio of two radiometric quantities as a function of wavelength."

A spectrophotometer is an instrument that uses a light source to measure the light absorption/transmittance and reflectance of the sample being measured. Each substance absorbs and reflects light back over a different wavelength. A black substance would absorb all light, a white substance would reflect all light, and all colors would fall in between, absorbing some light and reflecting light back at specified wavelengths. It is the reflected light that our eyes see. Industries that use specific colors for products commonly use spectrophotometry to match samples.[37] This technology is so precise, it can even tell the difference between extra virgin olive oil that comes from Italy and olive oil that comes from Spain.[38] Currently, we use spectrophotometry to analyze plants,[39] pharmaceuticals,[40] food,[41] and more.

From a scientific standpoint, energetic particles have a specific time, cycle, and duration as they move. Therefore, energy can be qualified and quantified. You may remember E=MC2. The energy of food and sunlight can be measured with a spectrophotometer. Consider that different colored wavelengths of light from the sun are more or less dominant at different times of the day, depending on the angle of the earth, the earth's atmosphere, and the position of the sun. Then consider the energy wavelength of a food or group of foods and connect it to the circadian rhythms of organs and systems, and you will get the basis for the 7X Method.

For the rest of us, let's make it simpler. We know the intensity of the sun's rays also changes throughout the day. On a summer day, we need sunblock around noon and into the mid-afternoon. This is when the sun's rays are the strongest. This is also when we are recommended to eat raw green vegetables and red meats; these foods are the hardest to digest. It all makes sense if you think about it.

It is hypothesized that for these metabolic processes and the needs of these local clock rhythms to be satisfied, the gut secretes digestive enzymes for that specific food group as dictated by central (SCN) and peripheral (each organ's) circadian rhythms.[42] In other words, we think that at different times of day, our body secretes digestive enzymes for specific types of food based on the energetic frequency of that food.[43] As I said, I no longer need to take digestive enzymes since starting this diet over two years ago, after taking digestive enzymes twice per day for almost 20 years. I hope that this book will inspire more research in this area. I think it's definitely worth investigating!

CHAPTER 4

Overview of the 7X Method

Now that you have a basic understanding of why you shouldn't be counting calories and macros and how circadian rhythms and quantum energy impacts your well-being, not only should you be feeling pretty smart, but you now have the foundation to understand the 7X Method.

The entire premise of this diet is the understanding that all systems of the body function in cycles: peak activity, nourishment, and rest/repair according to their individual circadian rhythms. Think about your muscles. When you work out, you stimulate the fibers and cells for peak activity. Then, after you work out, you nourish your body ideally with protein, and you have time to rest so the muscle can repair and build back stronger. Most people naturally understand this cycle of activity, fuel, and rest when it comes to optimizing muscles, so now we have to apply this understanding to all body systems.

With the 7X Method, foods are assigned an energetic value based on the discrete type of energy they contain. There are seven food groups based on the type of energy that a particular food has, which also corresponds to seven different types of energy that the body requires at specific times throughout the day.

Ideally, you would eat seven times per day, beginning around 7-8 a.m. and stopping by 6-7 p.m. You don't have to follow this perfectly to reap the benefits, but if you suffer from a chronic metabolic illness, you should adhere to this eating schedule as closely as possible. Here's a sample of what that would look like:

- **7-9 a.m.:** Coffee or tea, real dark chocolate (optional), nut/berry smoothie (optional), sunlight (preferred), exercise (ideal)

- **9-11 a.m.:** One piece of fruit or real, cold-pressed fruit juice (no mainstream brands or other pasteurized juices)

- **11 a.m. - 1 p.m.:** Green drink or smoothie and salad

- **1-3 p.m.:** Protein such as fermented foods, sprouted grains, red meat, or other animal product

- **3-5 p.m.:** Non-green veggies, i.e., carrot/ginger juice, V8, or you can drink a hot soup; dried papaya or mango

- **5-6 p.m.:** Kombucha, herbal tea, or a spoonful of peanut butter or hummus

- **6-7 p.m.:** Dinner with family consists of a small serving from the white foods group, green or non-green cooked vegetables (raw veggies have too much energy), light protein like fish or poultry (no red meat at dinner except on Friday)

I don't always get the seven food groups in every day, but on the days that I do, my mental clarity and physical energy are through the roof! So, this plan isn't about perfection; it's about having the tools and knowledge to organize your day for optimal nourishment and support of all the organs and systems in your body. Realistically, I want you to look at the clock when you sit down to eat and make sure you are getting something from the corresponding food group for that time period. Think of this like the periodic table of elements you learned about in grade school. You remember how the elements are categorized by their electric charge. Similarly, the foods in the charts below are categorized by their type of energy or electric charge.

1. Pulsating, Start-up Energy (Purple Food Group 7-9 a.m.)

2. Luminous, Light Energy (Blue Food Group 9-11 a.m.)

3. Kinetic, Propulsive Energy (Green Food Group 11-1 p.m.)

4. Thermic, Heat Energy (Red Food Group 1-3 p.m.)

5. Static, Steady Energy (Yellow Food Group 3-5 p.m.)

6. Magnetic Energy (Orange Food Group 5-6 p.m.)

7. Insular, Contracted Energy (White Food Group 6-7 p.m.)

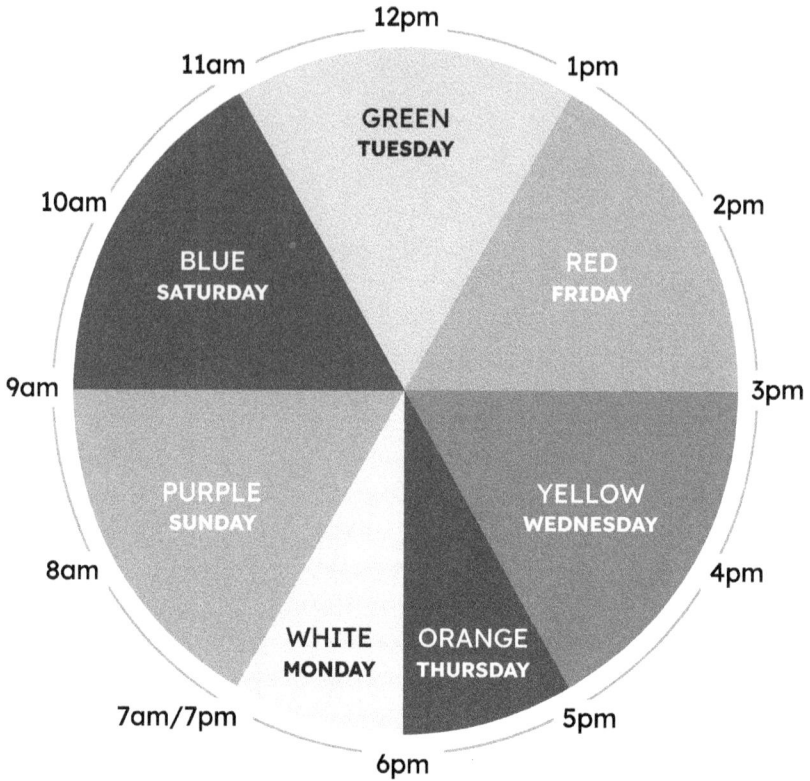

Purple Group	Nourishes in	Energetic Quality of Food Based on Fre-
7–9 a.m. Sunday -Electro-Pul- sating, Start- up Energy	Body, DNA repair and regeneration Pituitary and Pineal Gland	quency of Color to Align Endocrine System. Nuts, seeds, nut milks, black tea, matcha tea, coffee, honey, agave, stevia, monk fruit, REAL chocolate, cacao, royal jelly, coconut, peanuts/peanut butter, berries *Alternatively, you may continue your fast from the night IF you go outside and watch the sunrise; the sun activates this energy group

Blue Group **9–11 a.m.** Saturday Electrolumi- nous, Light Energy	Membranes, hyaluronic acid, eyes, thyroid	All fresh and dehydrated fruits, honeydew melon, figs, dates, prunes, blueberries, strawberries, raspberries, bananas, pitaya/ dragon fruit, dates, acai, pomegranate, pineapple, all cactus fruits, all tropical fruits, apple, starfruit, kiwi, pear, cantaloupe, papaya, mango, citrus fruits, cold-pressed juices (no mainstream or pasteurized brands)
Green Group **11 a.m.– 1 p.m.** Tuesday Electroinetic Energy	Skin, ears, genitals, nose tongue (sen- sory organs)	All green vegetables, cucumber, mint, cilantro, parsley, spinach, kale, watercress, celery, alfalfa, kelp, algae, broccoli, bok choy, artichoke, hearts of palm, broccoli rabe, escarole, arugula, grasses, sea kelp, spirulina, chlorella, blue-green algae, avo- cado, matcha tea powder, bananas
Red Group **1–3 p.m.** Friday Electrother- mic Energy	Blood, kid- neys, muscles, adrenals, heart	Proteins, all meat, lamb, bison, chicken, duck, beef, eggs, fish Fermented foods like miso, tempeh Germinated grasses, sprouted grains, nut and seed cheeses, mushrooms, whey pro- tein, dairy, beets, tart cherries/juice
Yellow Group **3–5 p.m.** Wednesday Electrostatic Energy	RNA repair/ regeneration, lungs	Squash, carrots, peppers, eggplant, av- ocado, ginger, turmeric, bamboo shoots, zucchini, olives, nightshades/lectins, sweet potato Vine vegetables: beans, peas, tomatoes Papaya, mango, cantaloupe, sweet potato, avocado, white potato
Orange Group **5–6 p.m.** Thursday Electromag- netic Energy	Digestive system, Liver Pancreas	Legumes, beans, tahini, lentils, edamame, peanuts, herbal tea
White Group **6–7 p.m.** Monday Electroinsular Energy	Bones Ner- vous System Thymus	Brown/jasmine/basmati rice, oats, white (older) coconut, white potatoes, jicama, cauliflower, quinoa, cassava, yucca, sweet/ green plantains, zucchini, corn, amaranth, rice milk, oat milk, gluten-free pastas, millet

CHAPTER 5

Purple, Blue, and Green Groups

THE PURPLE FOOD GROUP (7–9 A.M.)

The first group we are going to cover is the purple group, which is the group that contains electro-pulsating, or start-up, energy that assists with DNA repair and regeneration. And yes . . . coffee is in this group! So the foods in the purple group are stimulating. But, of course, you know that because so many Americans are addicted to their morning coffee.

At this time of the day, the pineal gland–which has been working all night long to create melatonin–is shutting down; but before it enters a stage of rest/repair, it needs nourishment from the purple group. Some examples of foods that belong in the purple group are nuts, seeds, berries, cacao, almond milk, cashew milk, macadamia milk, coconut milk, coffee (you may add honey, agave, stevia, or monk fruit), black tea, REAL dark chocolate (not processed with alkali), cacao, royal jelly, coconut, pea-nuts/peanut butter. Alternatively, you may continue your fast from the night IF you go outside and watch the sunrise; the sun activates this energy group.

Are you a morning coffee or tea drinker? Don't worry, this doesn't have to change. You can start your day with 1 cup of OR-GANIC coffee or tea, taken with MCT oil or nut milk if desired, ideally sweetened with honey, agave, monk fruit, or stevia. DO NOT use artificial sweeteners of any kind, as they are toxic. Toxins are stored primarily in fat tissue, organs, and bones.[44]

Here is an example of breakfast:

- Purple smoothie - made in a blender

- 8 ounces of coconut water

- 1/4 cup blueberries or blackberries

- 1/4 cup cranberries, dragon fruit, or other dark fruit like cherries, plums, figs, prunes

- 1/4 of a lemon

- Add 1 date only if extremely sour

- Mix and enjoy

This is the portion for one drink. If you want to meal prep for a few days, triple the ingredients. This smoothie is on the fancy side, but some people like fancy. I like simplicity. I usually use an entire liter of coconut water, one bag of frozen berries, and 1 cup of soaked almonds to make three portions, so I am prepped for the next couple of days. Tip: avoid using too much ice as it slows down the process of digestion and may cause stomach upset in some individuals, especially in colder climates. For athletes or those working hard physically, you may add more dates. They are used as a sweetener and are superior to sugar.

Honey may also be added as it has trace elements, minerals, and enzymes. Use coconut water as a base, if possible, or regular water. Avoid commercial store-bought juices because of the additives and sugars, including artificial sweeteners such as Splenda, Sweet & Low, Aspartame, Phenylalanine, high-fructose corn syrup, and modified cane sugar. This is also why coconut milk is a suitable base because it is high in fats, naturally sweet, and has no additives. You can also soak frozen cranberries, which are not sweetened; they make an excellent base for a smoothie. Experiment with different combinations.

There are several organic, non-GMO breakfast bars made of nuts that you can pick up from the supermarket, which makes it easy to run out the door to work. People with blood type A especially benefit from consuming nuts as a protein source.[45] There's a dark chocolate coconut bar made by a company called *Unreal* that I love. *Justin's* makes peanut, cashew, and almond butter cups and delicious nut butters. Sometimes, I grab a big piece of dark chocolate or a couple of spoonfuls of almond butter as I down my coffee.

Avoid breakfast bars containing grains as they do not support the endocrine system at this time of day. This includes granola since granola is mostly oats, which belong in the white group.

For persons with nut allergies or difficulty digesting nuts, you may incorporate darker berries into this time slot: figs, blueberries, blackberries, raspberries, pomegranate, goji berries, acai, cherries, cranberries, etc. We understand that polyphenols such as resveratrol found in these foods affect the peripheral circadian clocks in rats. Still, we need to know how these foods affect human circadian clocks, and if signaling pathways, specific metabolites, or micronutrients are causing these shifts.[46] We still have a lot to learn, but the moral of the story is: eat your purple berries in the morning or grab a pomegranate juice; we know it's good for you!

The serving size is up to you in any food group and generally depends on your daily activity and energy needs. Eventually, many of your "false cravings" for large amounts of certain foods will diminish, and your eating patterns will normalize. Initially, eat the portions you desire without feeling guilt or shame. Now, I realize this is the complete opposite of what you've been told your whole life. But the 7X way of eating is your body's way of getting the proper energetic nutrition that it may not have had for a long time. Therefore, do not restrict portions, at least for the first week. Your body knows what it needs, and we are asking it to make large cyclic and metabolic changes—so equip your body for the transformation!

For example, for about the first six months I was eating this way, my body wanted two to three 12 oz portions of the green drink I made for lunch, but now I only have one 12 oz green drink. I must have gone years without getting enough greens, and my body needed to compensate. Listen to your body and pay attention to its signals. When you eat like this for months, you feel the changes. It's incredible. *This is the total transformation that you have been searching for.*

WEEKLY RHYTHMS: PURPLE=SUNDAY

Now, not only will you eat from the purple group between 7–9 a.m., but if you look at the chart, you will notice that each food group has a corresponding day, which means you can eat from the purple group all day Sundays. This means your body craves more pulsating, start-up energy on Sundays for DNA regeneration, pituitary and pineal gland restoration. What does this mean? You can eat purple foods outside of this timeframe on Sundays, and they won't cause indigestion or inflammation. It's also the one day of the week that having coffee in the afternoon won't throw off your adrenal glands. It also means your body can better tolerate chocolate for dessert or berries in the afternoon on Sunday because it craves more foods with this specific frequency for the whole day. I feel best when I stick to the seven food groups seven times every day. But if I am at a family gathering on a Sunday afternoon, it's nice to know that I can "cheat" a little and have chocolate and coffee at 2 p.m. with them if I want to break some rules.

One of the main reasons I wrote this book was to find research supporting the principles of this way of eating in time. It doesn't exist yet, and I hope that will change because this way of eating has worked for everyone I know who has tried it. I found research that correlates chemicals from the foods in the purple group with the health of our DNA. Recent anti-aging science states that maintaining telomeres is critical to delaying the onset of age-related diseases.[47] Telomeres are unique DNA that protect the end of chromosomes from becoming frazzled or damaged.[48] Here's a perfect analogy: If your chromosomes are a shoelace, then telomeres are the plastic tip that keeps your shoelaces from unraveling. Likewise, telomeres keep your DNA from unraveling. Resveratrol and other polyphenols found in dark berries, grape skins, pomegranate, etc., are helpful in healthy DNA replication.[49] In a nutshell, no pun intended, eating from the purple group nourishes the DNA, so it is an excellent way to fight aging.

Conversely, suppose you have a work schedule where you don't wake up until after 9 a.m. on a regular basis. In that case, your body will lack the vital nutrition it needs for DNA regeneration achieved by receiving sunlight or eating or drinking foods from the purple food group between 7 and 9 a.m. When the master circadian clock is thrown off, it affects all the other peripheral clocks in your body. You may have heard about the clinical studies regarding night shift workers and their predisposition to cancers and other stress-related diseases.[50] As mentioned, obesity, insulin resistance, cardiovascular disease, and other signs of metabolic syndrome have been linked to circadian disruption in humans.[51]

BLUE FOOD GROUP (9-11 A.M.)

The blue food group provides electro-luminous light energy and should be eaten between 9–11 a.m. This is when your cell membranes, eyes, and thyroid need nourishment. T3 and T4 hormone levels peak in the morning and drop off between 10 a.m. and 4 p.m.,[52] so it would make sense that your thyroid needs nutrition between 9 and 11 a.m. Luminous energy is the known energy of light you can see and feel. You may have heard that light is measured in lumens–foods with luminous energy have the energy you can feel as soon as you eat it.

Some examples of food from this group are all fresh and dehydrated fruits, honeydew melon, figs, dates, prunes, blueberries, strawberries, raspberries, bananas, pitaya/dragon fruit, dates, acai, pomegranate, pineapple, all cactus fruits, all citrus fruits, all tropical fruits, apple, starfruit, kiwi, pear, cantaloupe, papaya, and mango. This list is not exhaustive. Water-bearing fruits are easily digested and can rapidly provide energy.

Now, if you are consistently fasting until 1 p.m., your DNA repair, thyroid, and eyes are affected, and your body can't make the hyaluronic acid it needs...which means accelerated aging! Yes, you heard it here first: Long-term intermittent fasting for 16 hours per day can lead to imbalance and disease of the metabolic systems. Surprise–the internet is full of misinformation.

Satisfying this group can be as simple as an apple or another piece of fruit. The idea here with the apple is to give you a reference point so you can begin to rethink how you identify foods. On other diets, some fruits (like melons) may have a higher glycemic index or are high in sugar and not recommended, especially for insulin resistance. However, this is different with the 7X Method. The purpose of eating the apple between 9 and 11 a.m. is to consume water-bearing fruit during this period to satisfy your body's need for a specific electric charge. I am using the apple as an example because it is low in acid and the most popular fruit globally. Other fruit can be added daily to provide variety and keep your transition exciting. Boredom kills most people's enthusiasm, and I want to offer many options so you can decide what works for your lifestyle and your taste. Eat what is in season. Try one of those overpriced, weird-looking fruits in the exotic fruit section.

"The Blood Type Diet" is controversial among the scientific community as it has little scientific validity due to a lack of studies. It is extremely difficult for researchers to obtain funding for food-based studies. It is much easier to get a pharmaceutical company to sponsor a drug study. I include information on the Blood Type Diet because, anecdotally, I have seen support for some of its claims. I met a naturopath in California who looked at live blood under a microscope and reported differences in agglutination of red blood cells before and after making dietary changes based on blood type. Agglutination means that the red blood cells stick together like a stack of donuts, making it difficult to transport enough oxygen to the body, causing the person to feel lethargic. Personally, I would retain water in my midsection for days after eating chickpeas, black beans, or edamame, even if I ate them at the right time. Then I eliminated these foods and opted for herbal tea 5-6 p.m. instead, and I had no more bloating.

So hey, if you follow the 7X Method, but something still makes you feel lethargic, look at the foods listed in the blood type diet charts. If eliminating these foods still doesn't help, take a food sensitivity test for IgG (IgE tests for anaphylactic reactions, and you don't need a test for that because the reaction is instantaneous).

Do some fruits upset your stomach?

Blood Type A	Oranges, bananas, mangoes, and papayas are not well tolerated; opt for grapefruit, kiwi, lemon, or pineapple instead. Cantaloupe and honeydew melons have high mold content and should be avoided.
Blood Type B	Type B people should avoid persimmons, pomegranates, and prickly pears; all other fruits are well tolerated, and pineapple can help digestion.
Blood Type AB	Type AB people do not tolerate oranges, bananas, mangos, and guavas, but grapefruit and lemons are beneficial; vinegar can irritate, and lemon juice is a great alternative.
Blood Type O	Cantaloupe and honeydew melons have high mold content and should be avoided. People with blood type O have more acidic stomachs and do not tolerate most citrus fruits or strawberries, as well as other blood types.

Adapted from D'Adamo D, Whitney C. Eat Right 4 You Blood Type. 2008

WEEKLY RHYTHMS: BLUE=SATURDAY

You will notice on the chart that the blue food group is labeled "Saturday." This means your body will optimize foods from this group throughout the entire day on Saturdays. What's better than fresh fruit in the afternoon on a beach day or by the pool? Possibly sangria loaded with fruits or prickly pear margaritas? Sometimes when I feel like I need a detox, I eat mostly fruits all day Saturday and a small dinner, according to the chart.

THE GREEN GROUP (11 A.M.–1 P.M.)

The green group provides electro-kinetic energy and should be eaten between 11 a.m. and 1 p.m. This is one of the most essential "electrical charges" to consume because most Americans do not eat enough green veggies on a daily basis. Some people maybe eat broccoli once a week, and many never eat salads. Some examples of food from this group are all green vegetables, cucumber, mint, cilantro, parsley, spinach, kale, watercress, celery, alfalfa, kelp, algae, broccoli, bok choy, artichoke, hearts of palm, broccoli rabe, escarole, arugula, grasses, sea kelp, spirulina, chlorella, and blue-green algae. These foods nourish the kidneys, skin, ears, and sensory organs. Leafy greens provide an important electrical quality for many systems but are especially beneficial to sensory organs like the ears, nose, tongue, skin, and genitals, according to the timed eating protocols I learned. I would love to see research proving this. We know leafy greens provide us with Vitamin C, Vitamin K, folate, potassium, magnesium, and calcium, and these all benefit our kidneys.

This one timing correction alone will give you a daily energy boost in the afternoon, and you won't need to rely on coffee for energy after lunch! This is often a neglected group of foods for those struggling to lose weight. I prefer to make green drinks, as I can get a lot of nourishment in my body quickly, and it digests more easily than a salad. You can also eat green salads if you prefer; either is fine. I recommend adding green drinks or smoothies, even if you have a salad for lunch, so your body gets sufficient kinetic energy to boost you through the early afternoon. When I have a green drink while sitting at my computer working, after about 15 minutes, I feel so energized that I have to get out of my chair and do something active. It's amazing!

You can make many variations from an abundance of green foods to make delicious drinks. For example, you can use coconut water as a base or water with an apple, kiwi, or pear. I like to make all of my drinks in a blender versus a juicer for several reasons: consistency; they tend to be a little thicker and a little more filling. I like the fiber in the drink, so I blend all my fruits and veggies in a blender. I typically add avocado and make it more of a smoothie; this helps me feel fuller for longer. You can add a banana to make it more filling. Vitamix works well and can cook your vegetables if you prefer soup in the cold winter months.

If weight loss is a goal or increasing the overall energy in the body is needed, this is one of the best habits to create. These drinks are not only nutritious, but they also are fast, delicious, and give a boost of energy mid-day. At the beginning of the program, it is permissible to use dates, honey, and apples as sweetness for those of you that have developed a sweet tooth from the Western diet. It is crucial to allow the body to slowly adapt its taste buds during this adjustment period. They will adjust over time. Don't force yourself to drink or eat something that tastes bad to you. Make this a go-to drink to help cleanse and revitalize your cells. You don't need copious amounts; in fact, it's better to start slowly. Even if you eat a salad for lunch, including a green drink will help flatten your tummy and increase energy levels. Here is one of my favorite green drink recipes:

Green drink, for an individual portion, combine the following:

- 1 green apple

- 1/4 cup cilantro

- 1/4 parsley

- 1 cup cucumber

- 1 cup fresh mint leaves

- A small wedge of lemon

- Coconut water

🔥 HOT TIP

Green drinks are readily available in the grocery store if you want them premade to save time. It's just way more expensive!

You can also make fresh green drink smoothies from powders. Adding cilantro and chlorella from green algae helps the body detox mercury. This is important if you eat a lot of sushi or have amalgam fillings in your teeth. Cilantro has also been shown to prevent lead accumulation in the body.[53] If you are one of those people with an aversion to the taste of cilantro, you can get this in supplement form, but fresh is best, of course. Fresh juices and blended drinks are of optimal value to your cells electrically.

You can swap out some of these greens for others or adjust amounts according to your taste. You will find a wide variety of these in the grocery store or farmer's market. As I mentioned, you can add avocado or banana to the green drink to make it more filling, and it won't disrupt the overall energetic charge of the drink. If you use orange juice as a base instead of water, this will change the flavor, and it can be a good change; however, you are starting to move away from the green spectrum foods, so avoid this as a routine and only do it once in a while as a treat. Sometimes we need a change, so do it, and don't feel guilty; don't make going away from the proper group a common occurrence. Remember, you can have water-bearing fruits all day on Saturdays without disrupting the program. I like to add frozen passion fruit cubes to my green smoothies on Saturdays.

🔥 HOT TIP

We all have busy schedules. Twice a week, I make juices and store them in the fridge. If you add lemon or lime juice as a preservative, they will be good for a few days. Mason jars are great because you can see what's inside and won't accidentally grab the wrong thing. Drinking fruit juice in the morning and vegetable juice around noon is easy.

Also, choose glass containers over plastic as plastic containers can contain phthalates and BPA, which are known endocrine disruptors and can be carcinogenic.[54] BPA in plastic water bottles has now been shown to bind to pancreatic islet cells, can cause impaired insulin or glucagon secretion, and lead to insulin resistance and possibly diabetes.[55] Yes, the toxins in plastic may also contribute to the rise in diabetes. Use stainless steel or glass when possible. Remove plastic storage containers and utensils in your kitchen, and use wood, bamboo, or stainless steel instead. Receipts are coated with BPA, so don't take them. Go electronic. If you search for "BPA and breast cancer," you will find a myriad of research articles linking plastics to cancer. It seems like we all know a woman who has had breast cancer. . . our goal is to reset our endocrine system and get our hormones balanced!

GREEN SALAD GUIDELINES

When you have a mixed greens salad, the best is to use olive oil dressing, and you can throw some tuna, chicken, or steak on this if you need more food or protein. We will get into the red group in just a bit, but yes, you can have protein anytime between 12-7 p.m. When it comes to green salads, you want to go easy on the mayonnaise and cut back on junk dressings like ranch or sugar-laden varieties. Instead, use simple condiments like mustard, hot sauce, or pickled foods, and avoid overprocessed foods like ketchup, mayonnaise, ranch dressing, and sugary barbecue sauce. A good guide for salads is the Mediterranean diet, which has been scientifically proven to improve health in clinical studies. So, choose options that are encouraged on the Mediterranean diet, which emphasizes whole foods and good fats, and order them according to the 7X Method of eating to maximize your health and energy!

When it comes to using oils in your diet, olive oil, avocado oil, and coconut oil are superior because they contain higher levels of omega-3. Many oils on the market are seed oils with higher levels of omega-6. Excessive intake of omega-6 fatty acids can contribute to inflammation because they more readily oxidize in the body, which is the opposite of what we want. Canola oil is garbage because of its high percentage of omega-6 fatty acids. Even sunflower and grapeseed oil are not good for you.

If you aren't in the habit already, make sure you read every label in the grocery store—and notice that sometimes, the most wholesome foods don't have labels! At first, this may seem time-consuming or cumbersome, but eventually, you will find your favorite brands readily available, and shopping will be a breeze. If you don't like the first coconut oil you try, you may like another type, such as filtered versus unfiltered or virgin vs. non-virgin.

Suppose you aren't a smoothie or salad person or don't live in a tropical climate like I do. In that case, you can do a broccoli stir-fry with protein (no rice for lunch or you will fall asleep), green veggie cakes, zucchini noodles with vegan pesto, asparagus, and shaved balsamic caramelized brussels sprouts are great for a change, or a cold climate! You can also steam spinach or oven-roast kale to decrease the oxalates. This is preferable over eating spinach and kale raw because research shows that vegetarians who consume more vegetables will have a higher intake of oxalates, which may reduce your body's calcium availability.[56] These oxalates can also lead to the development of gout and kidney stones.

Another great and simple option is to steam broccoli, put it into a blender with some bone broth or the water you cooked in, add salt, and then puree. This is very satisfying. If you need more substance, add avocado to make it creamier, and season it with nutritional yeast or aminos for a salty flavor. People with blood type A especially benefit from broccoli, kale, collard greens, and spinach. With type O, brussels sprouts and mustard greens can inhibit thyroid function, so if that's you or a family member, you may want to avoid these two veggies.[57] I have included recipes for soups in this book, including chunky soups with chicken or other proteins, like Colombian sancocho or borscht.

Salt is good because it conducts electricity. Use sea salt, Celtic salt, or Himalayan salt. Do not use iodized table salt, as it is stripped of nutrients and has no minerals. Instead, I add salt to my green juices to get more electrolytes to support the high level of activity that I subject my body to.

WEEKLY RHYTHMS: GREEN=TUESDAY

The green group is associated with Tuesday, meaning that your body likes more greens on this day. The kinetic energy of green foods nourishes the skin and sensory organs: ears, genitals, nose, and tongue. If you are extra hungry on a Tuesday, go for a snack with something green. Add some broccoli soup or steamed veggies to your evening meal. This would be a perfect evening for a green veggie stir fry (with rice) for dinner.

CHAPTER
6

Red, Yellow, Orange, & White Groups

RED FOOD GROUP (1–3 P.M.)

Foods from the red group provide electro-thermic energy, which nourishes the heart, kidneys, and adrenal glands. The goal is to specifically nourish these organs between 1 and 3 p.m. when the sun is at its highest point, and your digestion is optimal. This group of foods is comprised of both protein-based and fermented foods such as all meat, lamb, bison, chicken, duck, beef, eggs, fish, fermented foods like miso, tempeh, germinated grasses, sprouted grains, nut and seed cheeses, mushrooms, protein shakes, and whey protein. Red meat like beef, veal, bison, and lamb should be restricted to this time of day when the sun is in the highest position in the sky.

The red group is unique in that you can eat some foods from the red group on any day of the week after noon. You can layer easy-to-digest proteins such as sprouted grains, fish, or chicken on your salad at lunch or with dinner. Your body may need more protein than you can get by eating these foods only between 1 and 3 p.m., especially if you are blood type O. Protein helps you feel full in the afternoon.

Now, you may be wondering, "*Shouldn't I eat bacon and eggs for breakfast?*" Well, it's not ideal, and here is why: It all goes back to our circadian rhythm and the circadian rhythm of our adrenal glands. Earlier in this book, we learned that when we wake up in the morning, and the sun hits our eyes, the SCN stimulation in our brain triggers communication along the hypothalamic-pituitary-adrenal axis. The brain tells the adrenals that it's time to prepare for work. Then, thirty minutes after you wake up, your adrenals release a giant burst of cortisol to get you going for the day; this is called the *cortisol awakening response* (CAR).

Your cortisol levels at the CAR can be as much as 20 times your nighttime cortisol levels. According to the literature, this peak cortisol production is designed to happen 4–6 hours before increased eating activity,[58] which is right as we are getting into the timing for the red group.[59] The circadian rhythm of the adrenals is one reason why we aren't consuming meat or eggs for breakfast with the 7X Method; our body wants nourishment from these foods later in the day.

Between 1 and 3 p.m., your body benefits from 3-6 ounces of grass-fed beef, bison, lamb, fish, chicken, turkey, or as an alternate, fermented or vegetarian sprouted food. Use your best judgment and your own common sense; if you are a 6'2" male, you may need bigger portions than a 5'1" female. Also, if you are eating to optimize your health and maintain your body weight, you need bigger portions than if you are trying to lose weight.

All sprouted foods can be eaten in this time frame, which includes all sprouted grasses, such as wheatgrass or alfalfa, and sprouted grains, such as quinoa or rice. So let me be clear, you can digest rice or quinoa at this time of day without feeling sleepy, *only if it is sprouted*. When grains and seeds are sprouted, it changes their chemical composition and increases amino acid content to where you receive the same thermic charge that you would from eating animal protein.[60] You can use sprouted grain bread to make a sandwich if you like. You have to see what feels good with your body. You should feel energized after eating. If you feel lethargic after eating a particular food, then it's not right for you at that time of day, or perhaps not at all.

Aren't plant-based diets the best for everyone?

Blood Type A	Fermented foods like miso are an excellent alternative to meat consumption. In addition, people with blood type A have low stomach acid due to their agricultural ancestors; they benefit from avoiding meat and shifting to a more plant-based or pescatarian diet
Blood Type B	Shellfish should be avoided due to lectins that disrupt the type B system, but fish is a good staple protein. In addition, people with blood type B who suffer from fatigue or immune deficiencies should avoid chicken due to a lectin it contains, which can lead to strokes and immune disorders.

Blood Type AB	People with type AB should eat lamb, mutton, or rabbit in preference to turkey or beef and decrease animal fats in their diet due to their predisposition to have elevated blood cholesterol levels. Type AB also has low stomach acid and should decrease consumption of meats if trying to lose weight but can tolerate eggs and fish.
Blood Type O	Because people with blood type O have a more acidic stomach, fermented foods should be avoided. People with blood type O are the most primal, have the highest level of stomach acid, and need more animal protein than other blood types. Stick to 6 oz portions and increase the frequency of consumption between 12–6 p.m. as activity or stress levels increase.

D'Adamo D, Whitney C. Eat Right 4 You Blood Type. 2008.

Hard-boiled or deviled eggs could be a good snack here. It may be a big deviation from your normal routine and may seem inconvenient to follow this timing exactly. Still, you can do it for one week to reset your metabolism. You will realize that eating your biggest serving of proteins in the afternoon is much easier on your digestion than eating them for dinner. Raw nut cheeses are an excellent alternative to cow's milk products and do not produce any toxins after digestion unless there are nut allergies. Nut cheeses can be found in the vegan section of your local grocery store.

A portable snack for this time of day is:

- 2 hard-boiled eggs, or

- 3-6 oz fish (preferably fresh over canned due to histamine content of canned foods), or

- 3-6 oz nitrate-free sliced turkey, seasoned chicken breast, or grilled steak

It's no secret that omega-3 fatty acids are excellent for the heart, brain, and skin. You want to target a variety of DHA and EPA-based foods, so try to alternate the types of proteins you eat for omega-3 and 6 essential fatty acids. DHA omega-3 is found throughout the body and is most abundant in the heart, brain, and eyes. DHA is the component that helps the helps the cells of the brain, heart, eyes, and nervous system develop and perform properly through all stages of their growth.

Human cell membranes are approximately 75% fat and 25% protein,[61] depending on what type of cell they are, so the goal is to include these these foods at this time.

Avoiding greasy proteins and cheeses is also essential. Just say "No" to deep-fried animals. Eliminating pork is a good idea for many reasons, namely parasites such as Toxoplasma Gondii, Sarcocystis, Taenia, and Trichinella.[62] If you're not afraid of parasites, search the web for "neuroparasitology." You're welcome.

One last thing about the red group: If you are thinking, *"Who has time to eat meat between 1 and 3 p.m.?"* I don't want you to get super hung up on exact times and beat yourself up for not being perfect. Eating a salad with steak or chicken is ideal if you have a lunch meeting. However, eating that same steak salad after 7 p.m. will cause indigestion and inflammation. Sometimes I like to cook early dinners on weekends, especially when it's cold. Oven-roasted rosemary lamb with root vegetables is great for an "early bird special."

WEEKLY RHYTHMS: RED=FRIDAY

If you look at the food chart, you will see that the red food group also says Friday. What this means is that your body can better digest foods from this group throughout other times on this day. For example, you can have beet juice in your morning blend instead of restricting it to 1–2 p.m. Being part Italian, I'm a sucker for a good bolognese. I love having dairy/gluten-free potato gnocchi with bolognese and red wine for Friday night supper. It's not like you can never eat steak for dinner; save it for Friday. Friday evenings are also ideal for grilling burgers. If you are one of those people who complain about not being able to digest red meat, it's likely that you are just eating it at the wrong time. With the 7X Method, you will immediately notice a difference in your body's digestion. It's incredible!

YELLOW FOOD GROUP (3–5 P.M.)

The foods in the yellow group have more of a static energy property, so you won't get the energy boost from them that you do when you have a green drink at noon. These foods nourish the lungs and RNA repair and regeneration. Foods in the yellow group include non-green vegetables, root vegetables, nightshades/lectins, and all vine vegetables.

Now, let's go back to what we know about RNA regeneration. Remember the cortisol awakening response (CAR) that's activated around 7:30 a.m.? This cortisol secretion helps synchronize cells throughout the body with the external light cycle.[63] This process occurs primarily by the clock gene transcription.[64-66] Gene transcription is the process of copying a segment of DNA (a gene) into RNA. The RNA is eventually used as a template for protein synthesis. Clock genes exist in all cells, so your body is continuously replicating RNA to maintain the circadian rhythms in your body. Gene transcription occurs for all types of human DNA and RNA and is activated by the enzyme RNA polymerase. This enzyme is complex, but one of the main co-factors is magnesium. Magnesium is found in squashes, root vegetables, and onions. According to the timed-eating protocol, you need to eat non-green veggies between 3 and 5 p.m. to provide the right energy vital to this process.

Mom was right when she told us to eat our veggies! Please do what you can to get a dose of them in the late afternoon, at least a few days per week. For a snack, you can have a small carrot salad made from grated carrots with apple cider vinegar and a spray of coconut oil and salt. Tomato soup, split pea soup, steamed squash, and carrot and ginger soup are great options! Just steam carrots, add grated ginger, salt, bone broth, and a piece of garlic if desired. Put it in the Vitamix blender; it's done in minutes and great on a cold day or served chilled on a hot day-this makes a super easy solution to a light meal or early dinner. Sweet plantains make a great snack. This is also the right time of day to have carrot/beet/ginger juice. If you are on the go or unable to eat at this time due to work, grabbing pressed juice may be the best thing for you.

Mangos, some melons like cantaloupe, and papaya can also be eaten here in this time frame as they are in this group of yellow foods. Another snack option is plantain chips and guacamole. You may notice an overlapping in the timing of some foods. Certain foods and times have an overlap to them, like white potatoes, peanuts, bananas, or avocados. After some time and practice, you will get the hang of it.

Why do some vegetables make me bloated or give me heartburn when others can eat them without any problem?

Blood Type A	Avoid tomatoes. Corn should be avoided because it can affect insulin production, contributing to diabetes and obesity. Bell peppers, potatoes, and cabbage irritate the digestive tract and should be avoided. Fermented olives can also agitate the stomach lining.
Blood Type B	Tomatoes should be avoided, also avoid corn due to the type of lectin it contains.
Blood Type AB	Tomatoes are ok. Avoid corn due to the type of lectin it contains.
Blood Type O	Cabbage and cauliflower can inhibit thyroid function. Tomatoes are ok. The molds in shiitake mushrooms and fermented olives can trigger allergic reactions for blood type O. Corn should be avoided by those with blood type O because it can affect insulin production, contributing to diabetes and obesity.

D'Adamo D, Whitney C. Eat Right 4 You Blood Type. 2008

WEEKLY RHYTHMS: YELLOW=WEDNESDAY

The yellow food group can be efficiently digested on Wednesdays outside of its regular 3–5 p.m. time zone. My Wednesday dinner menus may include eggplant, tomato, peppers, green beans, or peapods. Who doesn't like (gluten-free) pasta prima-vera, chicken fajitas, or veggie stir fry?

My intention in sharing the "Weekly Rhythms" information is to allow you to have more leeway and freedom with your food so you don't feel so restricted. While adding more foods from the yellow group to your lunch or dinner on a Wednesday is unnec-essary, it may be more fun. If roasted eggplant or stuffed peppers are one of your favorite dinner meals, try making it on a Wednes-day when it digests better.

THE ORANGE FOOD GROUP (5–6 P.M.)

According to the timed eating protocols, the foods in the or-ange group have magnetic energy and can contribute to improv-ing digestion and resetting the pancreas in the setting of insulin resistance, but only when ingested within this timeframe, even in small amounts. This is the group that I am most interested in re-searching further. A nurse practitioner worked at an endocrinol-ogy clinic in the Midwest a few years ago. Many of her patients had diabetes and had continuous glucose monitoring, meaning they had a device implanted on their bodies to give frequent, real-time blood sugar readings. She asked some of the patients to follow this diet loosely, and they reported needing to use less insulin. Insulin is an expensive drug, and if diabetic patients can use less of it by following this diet, it could be huge for our health-care system. Unfortunately, that nurse practitioner moved on to another position, so I cannot get any more data from her patients other than the anecdotal evidence described here.

This group contains lentils, all beans, and legumes. More research needs to be done on how these foods affect blood sugar regulation when taken at precisely this timeframe. The liver repairs at night, which implies that it works during the day and needs nutrition at the end of the day around 5–6 p.m.[67] Have just a spoonful of hummus or peanut butter if you don't feel very hungry at the time. Mint tea, chamomile, lemon grass, or other herbal tea can be added to or taken as an alternative to food; these are aromatic plants and digestives. The goal is to give your body the specific electric charge that it requires.

Quick snacks from this group might include:

- Lentil soup or hummus (with carrots and celery from the yellow food group if eaten at 5 p.m.)

- Herbal tea or kombucha (especially if Blood Type O)

- A spoonful of peanut butter (because peanuts are technically legumes)

Many Americans experience indigestion, bloating, and water retention after eating beans and legumes. However, that's often because beans and legumes are consumed at the wrong time of day. I am blood type O and so are almost 40% of Americans,[68] which means beans and legumes equal indigestion, bloating, and water retention. If I am hungry, I'll take a spoonful of peanut butter, but usually, herbal tea or kombucha at this time is perfect for my appetite. And while the Latin culture may be good about getting beans in their diet, eating beans with rice doesn't exactly follow the 7X Method unless you eat them closer to 6 p.m. Lentils can be made into soups and seasoned with herbs, nutritional yeast, or miso. There are many Indian recipes for these lentils and beans, far too many to mention here, so experiment and have fun. Find what works for you.

Lentils are a great source of short-chain fatty acids, which are produced when the fiber is fermented in the colon, thus providing a source of energy for the colon. In addition, the microbial metabolites (acetate, propionate, butyrate) formed in the fermentation process directly affect circadian clock gene expression within the liver cells.[69] Short-chain fatty acid receptors have also been found in adipose (fat) tissue and pancreatic islets.[70] Eating legumes or drinking tea between 5 and 6 p.m. is often the most challenging change for people to make; I know it was for me!

Studies have shown that the pancreas has a distinct circadian rhythm, with insulin secretion being highest in the morning and decreasing throughout the day. Remember, you don't need a large quantity of food from this food group, but you do need the electrical charge given by this food because it switches on the pancreas when taken at this time only. This is thought to be true because several liver enzymes that are involved in sugar metabolism, including fructose metabolism, glycolysis, and the citric acid cycle, are also under circadian control.[71] This pattern helps regulate glucose metabolism, providing the body with energy to meet the demands of the day, and promoting relaxation and rest at night.

Why can some people tolerate eating beans and others can't?

Blood Type A	Benefits from proteins contained in this group except for garbanzo beans/chickpeas, kidney, lima, and navy beans, which have a lectin that decreases insulin production.
Blood Type B	Avoid lentils, beans, and peanuts.
Blood Type AB	They can tolerate lentils and peanuts and benefit from proteins contained in this group except for garbanzo beans/chickpeas, kidney, lima, and navy beans, which have a lectin that causes a decrease in insulin production.
Blood Type O	People with blood type O do not metabolize beans and legumes that well and may benefit from having an herbal tea at this time frame instead.

D'Adamo D, Whitney C. Eat Right 4 You Blood Type. 2008

WEEKLY RHYTHMS: ORANGE=THURSDAY

The orange food group falls on a Thursday. It is crucial to the vitality of the digestive organs, liver, pancreas, cells, and cell membranes. This is the most important group for people with diabetes to consume at the right time daily because anecdotal evidence suggests it resets the pancreas's circadian rhythm. Research is underway, although data has yet to be published. Stay tuned for the revolution in blood sugar regulation! In the meantime, you can enjoy going to the Israeli restaurant down the street and picking up shawarma with hummus to go (no pita=no bloating)–such a treat!

THE WHITE GROUP (6–7 P.M.)

Foods from the white group provide electro-insular energy, which is inward and calming to the nervous system. This means they are the last food group to be eaten because they have an energetic quality that helps you wind down. These foods nourish bones and the nervous system. Some examples are brown/jasmine/basmati rice, oats, white (older) coconut, sweet potato, white potatoes, jicama, cauliflower, quinoa, cassava, yucca, sweet/green plantains, zucchini, corn, amaranth, cereals, oatmeal, rice milk, oat milk, and gluten-free pasta.

The foods in this group are primarily carbohydrates and of grain origin. We want to focus on foods with the most regenerative potential. Choosing yucca, potato, millet, or oatmeal can be considered more optimal than white flour products. These foods reduce nerve stimulation and prepare the body for sleep, which is why they are often referred to as comfort foods. They may often make people feel tired, especially after consuming them outside of this time frame. White foods have a very dominant electric charge. After 6 p.m. is the only time white foods are efficiently processed. How often have you seen a coworker grab a coffee after having pasta or rice at lunch?

I know what you're thinking, *Carbs at night? Isn't that going to make me fat?* This is hard for people to believe, but *this* is the time to eat all those comfort foods! First, let me say that certain white foods are superior energetically to others, and this should make sense. For example, whole organic brown rice is superior to white pasta noodles even though they are both in the white food group. You must use your discretion when consuming white foods IF YOU WANT TO LOSE WEIGHT. But this is the time to eat white foods (carbs), but please decrease the amounts and choose the most nutritious whites. Bread and pasta are to be eaten very sparingly on special occasions for the weight conscious.

Interestingly, a study was done on 78 obese police officers who were given a diet that included white foods to be eaten only at night. After 180 days, it was observed that hunger and satiety scores were 13.7% higher in individuals consuming carbohydrates only at dinner, indicating that subjects were more satiated than in week one of the diet. They also had a greater reduction in BMI and waist circumference. In contrast, the control group, who received carbohydrates at every meal, reported a 5.9% lower hunger and satiety score compared with baseline.[72] It has been proven that a small serving of foods from the white group eaten only at dinner decreases abdominal fat.

A good example would be:

- Oven-roasted potatoes with herbs and olive oil; add rotisserie chicken if feeling starved or trying to gain muscle.

WEEKLY RHYTHMS: WHITE=MONDAY

You will see that the white food group corresponds with Mondays. God Himself must have known that Mondays would be crazy and that we would crave comfort foods and carbs! Monday is the day your body can efficiently digest the white foods outside the designated time. So, on Mondays, you can have rice or potatoes at lunch and not feel as tired afterward. I love cooking with *Andean* brand quinoa pasta or *Jovial* brand brown rice pasta.

Potato soup (dairy-free), baked potato (no sour cream, and use butter sparingly if you're trying to lose weight), or broiled red potatoes with fresh dill or parsley are good options. You can add small amounts of seasoning and nutritional yeast to give them a salty flavor. You can also add *Bragg* Amino Acid mix.

I advise my clients to avoid dairy products (except for grass-fed butter) during the first six months of being on the diet to decrease inflammation. This is especially true for people with blood types O or A who don't metabolize dairy well, women who are trying to re-calibrate their hormones, or those trying to reduce body fat. Cows are almost always pregnant. A 1,500-pound cow produces milk with enough growth hormone to sustain an 80-pound calf–that's literally 10 times the size of a human! Dairy products can be reintroduced to the diet slowly and eaten sparingly on a long-term basis. Cheese is not meant to be eaten every day. Generally, blood types AB and B tolerate dairy products better than type A or O, but there are always exceptions.[73]

CROSSOVER IN GROUPS

Now that you understand the color groups, please be aware that some foods have two kinds of energy. For example, avocados can be in the green group or the yellow group, but you can see this when you slice it open–two colors. Same thing with a zucchini: it's green on the outside so that it can be in the green group, but it's white on the inside so that it can go in the white foods group also. Potatoes (all varieties) can be in the yellow group because they are a vegetable, but they can also be in the white foods group because they have a calming energetic charge.

Now, what about peanuts? Do they belong to the purple group because they are nuts? Or are peanuts a legume belonging to the orange group? It's somewhat controversial, but I prefer to place them in both categories. Peanuts are not a great food in general because they are prone to having aflatoxins, a family of toxins produced by mold, which are known to increase the risk of liver cancer.[74] However, sometimes, if I am on the go or stuck in my car, a little packet of peanut butter is the easiest way for me to get the charge my pancreas needs between 5–6:00 p.m. Hence, you have to do your best and know that every step is progress!

Exercise, Weight Loss, and the **7X** Lifestyle

Not only is when you eat and what you eat important, but the quality of what you eat is equally so. If you want to decrease body fat, you have to stop eating toxins. The body uses fat cells to store toxins and keep them away from vital organs, so if your diet is laden with processed foods, chemicals, and additives, you will put unnecessary added stress on your body. Again, we are not concerned with calorie counting here, but we are interested in the specific electrical quality of the food and the time you eat it. You may also have a piece of "real chocolate." That means cacao or dark chocolate, not chocolate bars processed with alkali from a large corporation with genetically modified soy lecithin or milk ingredients.

Your morning coffee *must* be organic because coffee is one of the food products most heavily drenched in pesticides.[75] These pesticides are neurotoxins and xenoestrogens (estrogen-mimicking) that cause leaky gut or damage to the intestinal lining.[76] Conventional coffee is often contaminated with mold; the mycotoxin biproducts[77] from the mold are harbored in our liver. The more toxins accumulate in your liver, the less time it has to detox your hormones and perform other vital functions. (This is where some milk thistle or silymarin would be handy.)

If you aren't one of those people who wakes up starving or feels nauseous at the thought of eating breakfast, you may be able to skip the berries and nuts in this group and stick to coffee with MCT or nut milk as you start the program. This morning aversion to food is usually due to cortisol dysregulation (stress affecting your adrenal glands) and will normalize with time as you stick with the program. An alternative is to take hot water with honey and apple cider vinegar; this will give you the electric charge that your body needs. Eventually, your tastes and appetite will change, and you will enjoy eating nuts, chocolate, or berries between 7-9 a.m.

Suppose your schedule permits that you exercise in the morning before eating breakfast (you can have coffee/nut milk or honey/hot water/apple cider vinegar, so you aren't on a completely empty stomach). In that case, it will stimulate more growth hormone and activate the cortisol burst consistent with a healthy daily cortisol pattern.[78] If you tend to lean toward hypoglycemia, I do not recommend morning exercise before eating. Instead, eat something, even if it's just a handful of berries or a small piece of chocolate and coffee or tea with nut milk.

If you continue your fast through 9 a.m., ensure you eat something from the blue group between 9 and 11 a.m. Do not wait until noon to consume calories. A study on college-aged women showed that women who fasted until 12-1 p.m. did not have lower body fat or BMI, but skipping breakfast was associated with constipation, and menstrual irregularities.[79] Constipation, weight gain, and menstrual irregularities are all symptoms of an underactive thyroid. Eating water-bearing fruits between 9 and 11 a.m. nourishes the thyroid. Do you see the important connection between food and function?

Why else do we want to try to exercise in the morning shortly after waking up? According to research, morning exercise is best for the metabolism. For example, in mice, exercising upon waking enhanced 24-hour rhythms of skeletal muscle genes and metabolites related to carbohydrate metabolism, but exercise around bedtime negated these rhythms.[80] Mice sleep during the day and are active at night, which is obviously the opposite of humans, so it is not like comparing apples to apples. But it is interesting to note that exercising after waking up was shown to help the mice metabolize carbohydrates better, but exercising before bedtime was detrimental to carbohydrate metabolism.

Try this morning exercise before breakfast for seven days to jump-start your weight loss goals and shift your hormones in a more favorable direction. Naturally, this will increase cortisol levels. However, many of my coaching clients' test results show Stage 1 or Stage 2 adrenal fatigue, which means the adrenal glands are "tapped out" due to prolonged stress and can no longer secrete enough cortisol in the morning. Therefore, stimulating a burst of cortisol with high-intensity activity will help restore the normal pattern. Anecdotally, I can say adrenal fatigue is prevalent in our society, as I have seen in my clients' test results. A week of "exercise for breakfast" can help reset the diurnal cortisol pattern.

You can maintain this morning-exercise-for-breakfast routine as a long-term lifestyle. Be careful not to cause hypoglycemic episodes because this causes stress to the body. A five-year study showed that skipping breakfast was closely associated with annual increases in BMI and waist circumference among men, but eating breakfast more than four times per week may prevent excessive weight gain associated with skipping breakfast.[81] Again, please make sure to eat from the purple or the blue group after your fast, do not wait until the green group at noon.

A little stress is good. Too much stress is bad. Marathon runners subject their bodies to such high stress levels that it can lead to unbalanced hormones and low testosterone in men; I've seen it clinically. Most people would assume that marathon runners would be healthier than all of us, but it's often not the case. In "Pillar #1" of my book, *The THIN Formula*, I focus extensively on stress, cortisol, and melatonin. It's imperative to rebalance the diurnal curve with interval training or HIIT (high-intensity interval training) exercise 3-5 mornings per week, speak consistent positive affirmations throughout the day, and do daily three-minute meditations. These are some great lifestyle modifications to start with.

What is high-intensity interval training (HIIT), and why does it need to be done in the morning? High-intensity exercise is any activity that causes your heart rate to reach maximum levels (roughly 220 beats per minute–age) for a short period and then drop back down to an intensity where you can catch your breath. You continue this for about 20 minutes. I recommend this for men with low testosterone (less than 500 ng/dL) and men and women with low morning cortisol levels associated with adrenal fatigue. Cortisol levels are best analyzed through saliva, similar to the popular at-home DNA tests. Cortisol levels can be tested by spitting into a tube at four specific times in one day to obtain the diurnal pattern. The goal is to have intense morning exercise to raise your cortisol levels and mimic the diurnal pattern. By morning, I mean that you are done by 8 a.m. at the latest. You don't want a spike in cortisol at 11:00 a.m. Exercising after work or before dinner is a good time for HIIT also. Studies show that our coordination is better in the late afternoon.[82]

Conversely, you want evening activity to be lower in intensity because a spike in cortisol after dinner will delay your 9 p.m. release of melatonin. I personally do interval training three mornings per week to support my adrenal glands and then yoga two evenings per week as a part of my mental health and physical flexibility maintenance program.

Also, those with blood type O tend to benefit most from intense exercise.[83] As a rule of thumb, if you can continue exercising beyond 30 minutes, your routine is not intense enough to be considered HIIT. Less is more. Even a 15-minute HIIT will do the trick. We want to stimulate muscle growth with targeted exercise at a time in the day when growth hormone is elevated. You don't need much exercise when adhering to the 7X Method.

Interval Training is less intense than HIIT; the activities involve switching between moderate-intensity and low-intensity exercises. You can tell you are doing interval training if you are able to work out for 30-45 minutes. If you are new to working out, it may be better to start with interval training and then progress to HIIT. If you have an *Orange Theory* fitness facility near you, this is a great way to start because you can see your intensity on the television screens throughout the entire workout session and compete with yourself week after week. With some practice, you will become more aware of your body and be able to differentiate between interval training and HIIT. I see many of my female friends on social media posting their *Beachbody Fitness* morning workouts; this is great for moms because they can do it at home. The X3 Method with Dr. John Jaquish is great for men.

If you love yoga or Pilates, I don't want you to give that up. But please understand that these low-intensity activities are best done in the afternoon or evening when your cortisol levels are naturally declining. You aren't going to lose weight and reset your hormones by doing Pilates or jumping onto the elliptical for an hour in the morning. If the morning is the only time of day that you can schedule exercise due to work or family obligations, then keep the Pilates twice a week, but you must incorporate HIIT the other three days.

Our ancestors were hunters and gatherers, meaning they were most active around dawn and dusk.[84] If you can only exercise after dinner, you are technically following our inherited circadian clock. Just remember to keep the intensity low to moderate at this time, which means you can do interval training for 30-45 minutes or low intensity for 45-60 minutes.

Be careful not to train too hard and push your limits at this time in the evening because it will cause a physiological stress response and spike cortisol levels. For this reason, we also do not want to exercise after 9 p.m. because it interferes with melatonin release and can cause delayed-onset sleep. Remember, this master circadian rhythm of our sleep-wake cycle sets the pace for the circadian rhythms of all our organs and systems.

If you are not currently in the habit of exercising, consider beginning this program with the diet only. Then, after two weeks of adhering to the diet, you may start walking 30 minutes per day. You may continue walking daily for weeks 3-6, and by week 7, you will progress to interval training. One easy way to implement a 30-minute interval training program is by walking for two minutes and jogging for one minute. Then you repeat this cycle 10 times for 30 minutes total. Continue this for two weeks.

By the 3rd month (week 9), you should be able to incorporate 20 minutes of HIIT 2-3 times per week. I like to do this by walking for a couple of minutes, jogging for 3-5 minutes, and then sprinting as long as I can. I repeat this cycle 3-5 times, depending on how I feel that day. Usually, it's 15-25 minutes in total. Then I stretch. An alternative would be to search YouTube for a 20-minute home fitness routine that incorporates air squats, lunges, burpees, abdominal exercises, planks, etc.

The purpose of the exercise is not for weight loss. You can lose weight by eating the 7X Method without exercising. The purpose of exercise performed at specific times is to support your circadian clock, your organs, and your systems as part of the 7X Method.

Don't forget to schedule one day of rest. God said to remember the Sabbath to keep it holy and nourish your body by allowing it to recover. Nourish your spirit by giving gratitude for your blessings because if you are reading this right now, you are blessed to have the luxury of incorporating things into your life that extend beyond basic survival.

The ultimate goal of the 7X Method is to move beyond your current perception of food and create a functional lifestyle. Once you have your body communication systems integrated and the endocrine system functioning properly, you will be able to shift your focus away from the food obsession-deprivation model and enjoy all the diversity life has to offer. Remember, it's about *changing* your relationship with food. You can always eat what you want; you just have to wait for the right time of day to eat it!

CHAPTER 8

Getting Started: The 7-Day Nutrition Reset

The 7-Day Nutrition Reset is your kickstarter program to the 7X Method, and it's designed to reset your metabolic systems. Yes, you can have tremendous results in as little as seven days. To do this, you will eat seven small meals each day within a 10 to 12-hour window.

Who needs to do the 7-Day Reset? Anyone with an autoimmune disease, including diabetes, obesity, and cancer, should follow the strict timing for a minimum of seven days; because if you think about it, all of these health concerns result from a communication breakdown among the body systems. By eating out of these seven food groups at specific times of the day, you will realign the seven different energy groups in your body and reestablish the balance of brainwave frequencies, enhancing your ability to concentrate.

I recommend that anyone with digestive discomfort, autoimmune issues, or chronic pain give the 7-Day Reset a 100% effort. However, if you miss a mealtime, skip it and move on to the next time slot. Eventually, you will know what your body likes and needs, and naturally, you will create a balanced program that is unique to you and fits your lifestyle and needs, but here are some basics:

1. Have your first meal between 7-9 a.m., after sunrise.

2. Don't eat after sunset. Sure, we all have to make exceptions for meetings, dinner parties, etc., but don't make it a daily habit. Eating at night is the worst thing you can do to sabotage weight loss and hormone balance, specifically insulin, cortisol, and melatonin. If you live in a climate where the days are shorter during the winter months, it is understood that dinner at 6 p.m. will occur hours after sunset . . . these are guidelines, not hard rules! But if you can eat dinner at 5 p.m. instead of 6 p.m. in the winter months, it will help your energy levels stay at optimal levels.

3. Have nothing but water for at least 12 hours per day (when you aren't eating). Your liver is the only organ that processes hormones, and it needs a break from processing your food intake in order to manage your endocrine system, including your thyroid. For example, take your last bite of food at 7:30 p.m. and don't eat again until 7:30 a.m. Don't stress yourself out about exact times, but you get a general idea; don't

have coffee or eat breakfast at 6 a.m. and then eat dinner at 9 p.m., it's too much stress on your pancreas and liver. Try not to eat after 7 p.m. because it increases your insulin resistance, leading to belly fat. Eating a piece of pie at 8 p.m. has a similar effect on your insulin as if you ate two pieces of pie at 4 p.m. Your body is designed to release melatonin around 9 p.m. but if you eat food or have a glass of wine after 9 p.m. that delays the melatonin release because it turns your pancreas back on for insulin to be released and blood sugar to get into your cells. Our grandparents were really onto something with their "early bird special."

4. It's essential to not eat within two hours of going to bed. But don't go to bed with your stomach borderline growling either; otherwise, you will likely wake up at 4 a.m. from hypoglycemia. Hypoglycemia is stressful for the body and causes the adrenals to release cortisol because your body wants you to wake up and eat, so the hypoglycemia goes away. You want that burst of cortisol to occur around 7:30 a.m., not 4 or 5 a.m.! Find the sweet spot.

5. If you consistently fast until 1 p.m. your DNA repair, thyroid, and eyes are affected, and your body can't make the hyaluronic acid it needs. Hyaluronic acid occurs naturally in the skin by binding water to collagen to keep us looking young. Long-term intermittent fasting for 16+ hours will cause certain organs and systems to miss the nourishment they need at specific times routinely. Over time,

this can lead to imbalance and disease of the metabolic systems. The internet is full of misinformation about intermittent fasting and time-restricted eating.

6. Cooked green and non-green vegetables can be added to your white foods at dinner; raw green vegetables at dinner may give you difficulty sleeping due to their kinetic energetic quality. You can layer easily digestible proteins into other groups, like chicken on salad for lunch or fish with rice for an early dinner if you are feeling overly hungry or trying to build lean muscle mass. Avoid eating a big dinner on a regular basis. It's okay to be a little hungry when you go to bed; you will sleep better if your body is not busy digesting food.

7. Remember this point: If you want to reduce body weight, you must plan on reducing the volume of food after week one. Take the first week to adjust to shuffling foods around. Don't ever let yourself go hungry or feel starved or deprived.

8. When it comes to following the meal plan, I tried to create options for each time based on the most common food allergies or food sensitivities. Feel free to substitute based on your preferences but remember to update the grocery list accordingly. Many of the recipes make several portions so you can freeze the soups to eat them over the course of a few weeks instead of eating the same thing three days in a row. Don't get bored.

9. You may notice that there are no cow's milk products. Many of my clients need to rebalance their hormones. Cows are always pregnant; their hormones are passed through their "breast milk," and their hormones affect your hormones even if the label says "organic" or "no-added hormones." Many of my clients, including myself, have noticed immediate flattening of their tummies after taking milk and cheese out of their diet. Casein, the protein found in dairy products, lights up the same part of the brain as drugs do. Cheese stimulates dopamine production. It's okay to break up with cheese. It's a toxic relationship!

10. You may also notice that there are no wheat/barley/rye gluten-containing foods. The wheat we eat today is not like the wheat that our grandparents ate. It's been genetically modified for mass production. According to some sources, it contains up to 5X more gluten in it today than it used to. Gluten is the protein in wheat, and it closely resembles proteins found in our body structures, particularly the thyroid. Gluten is linked to Hashimoto's thyroiditis. Today's gluten has been shown to cause temporary interstitial permeability (Also known as leaky gut) in every human every time they eat it.[85]

Zonulin is a protein that regulates the permeability of tight junctions in the cells to the small intestine. Think of your gastrointestinal tract as an exclusive nightclub, and zonulin is like a security guard for your stomach lining, then comes along "gluten," the hot underage girl with a fake ID, to get into the club. This is kind of what happens every time you eat a croissant; the gluten tricks the zonulin into opening the tight junctions of the stomach lining, allowing undigested food particles to enter the bloodstream. When this occurs, the body reacts to the toxic invaders (undigested food particles) by creating an inflammatory response. This is essentially an immune reaction, and the symptoms present differently for different people. According to the Institute for Functional Medicine, people without celiac disease report gluten sensitivities that manifest as abdominal pain, bloating, altered bowel function, fatigue, headache, joint or bone pain, mood disorders (especially in children), and skin manifestations such as rashes or eczema. Your gut lining is about as thick as tissue paper, so it doesn't take much gluten to penetrate it.

The gut-brain axis connects the stomach and brain. The gut-brain axis is the two-way communication between the gut and the brain. This communication occurs through multiple pathways that include hormonal, neural, and immune messengers. The messages passed along this axis can begin in the gut, originate in the brain, or occur in both.[86] Research shows that the microbiota participate in signaling to maintain normal gut function and appropriate behavior, among other things.

Getting rid of gluten and dairy was a big help for me; almost all the joint pain in my hands and knees that I had previously attributed to "normal aging" went away. I still eat grass-fed butter, albeit sparingly, because that doesn't have the lactose (sugar) or casein (protein) that milk products have. Gluten is tricky because the antibodies stay in your blood for up to three weeks, so you really have to be strict with avoiding all wheat products all the time to reap the health benefits. But it's so worth it. Once you feel all your pains go away, you don't want them to come back.

If you have a leaky gut, you have a leaky brain. If toxins are leaking through your gut lining into your bloodstream, those toxins may also be crossing the blood-brain barrier into your brain. Do you ever feel really spaced out or sleepy after eating? This may be due to toxins leaking into your brain. Do you ever feel restless or have trouble sleeping? A leaky gut can also allow the release of fragments of gastrointestinal hormones into the brain, particularly CCK4 which can even cause anxiety and panic attacks.[87]

A leaky gut has been linked to autoimmune diseases such as multiple sclerosis, rheumatoid arthritis, celiac disease, inflammatory bowel disease, ankylosing spondylitis, cancer, autism, chronic fatigue syndrome, and more.[88] I don't know about you, but it's not worth eating a bagel or pizza if it's putting me at risk for these awful diseases.

Dairy and gluten; are they really that bad for everybody?

Blood Type A	Avoid wheat gluten, dairy, and eggs.
Blood Type B	Gluten inhibits insulin function, so avoid the gluten found in wheat. Can benefit from moderate consumption of dairy.

Blood Type AB	Avoid gluten found in wheat but can benefit from moderate consumption of dairy. However, African Americans or Asians with blood type B may have intolerances to dairy because, historically, there were no cows in Africa or Asia.
Blood Type O	Gluten inhibits insulin function. Avoid grains and dairy. African Americans with blood type O may want to avoid eggs also.

D'Adamo D, Whitney C. Eat Right 4 You Blood Type. 2008

DEBUNKING MYTHS:

1. Eating fat does not make you fat. Your brain is made of fat. All your nerves are covered in a fatty protective coating called myelin. You need good fats in order to have adequate sex hormones. With the help of bile from the gallbladder, your liver processes dietary fat into LDL cholesterol. LDL cholesterol, yes, the "bad cholesterol" is the building block of cortisol and all your sex hormones. LDL combines with vitamin B5 and an enzyme to make the precursor to cortisol, estrogen, progesterone, testosterone, etc. We need cholesterol in our skin cells to make vitamin D from sunlight. Having listened to many lectures, anecdotally I can tell you that most functional medicine or integrative health providers desire their patients to have serum vitamin D levels around 50,000. What are your levels?

2. No more carbohydrate shaming! Eating fruits at the right time is essential to your health. You can't just pop a multivitamin and expect to get the same nutrients as eating whole foods with actual plant-based micronutrients. The 7X Method is not about macro or micronutrients; it's

about getting the correct electric charge at the right time of day. Also, we need to permit ourselves to eat white foods as long as they are not processed. It's okay to eat a small serving of white food at night. It's not about calories or macronutrients. We must delete that file in our brains and reprogram our thinking. It's about a specific food with specific energy to nourish a specific system. It's all about timing!

3. The "body positivity" trend is dangerous if we normalize obesity, metabolic syndrome, and diabetes. Many people don't realize that when you gain body fat, there is an increase in metabolic demand on the heart, kidneys, liver, and the rest of your organs. When people gain weight, they grow bigger, but their organs don't. According to Johns Hopkins Medicine, there is a 30% increase in developing heart failure for every 5-unit increase in body mass. So, if your BMI (body mass index) was 25 ten years ago, and now it is 30, you have a 30% higher risk of developing heart failure. Similarly, if your BMI is 35, then you have a 60% increase in developing heart failure than you did 10 years ago.

4. Wolff's Law pertains to bones and essentially states that bones in a healthy animal will adapt to stresses or loads placed on it by becoming stronger as they go about their normal remodeling process. As a physical therapist, I can tell you that even osteoporotic women in their 60s and

70s would benefit from weight-bearing activity. This can be achieved by walking, using the elliptical to protect your knees or even resistance training with weights and bands. You are the creator of your body. When you provide the proper stimulus, you can change your physical being.

5. Holten's Curve is used by physical therapists, athletic trainers, and personal trainers to guide exercise programs. This theory pertains to building muscle. Muscles have different fibers that perform various tasks. You can use resistance training to make your muscles do different things. It is more complex with regard to the number of sets and the time taken to rest between sets, but let me break it down for you in the simplest way I can.

- If you want to increase circulation, you lift a very light weight or band 30+ reps.

- If you want to increase muscular endurance and lengthen the muscle, you train 13-25 reps using a light weight.

- If you want to make your muscles bigger and stronger, you lift a moderate weight of 8-12 reps.

- If you want to focus on increasing strength but not necessarily getting bigger, then you lift heavy weights for 3-7 reps.

- If you want to lift to increase power, you use a very heavy weight for 1-3 reps.

For those who want to gain muscle, you can add food from the red group (proteins) at lunch, dinner, and throughout the afternoon. Protein shakes at breakfast will inflame you, and you can't get shredded when your body is in an inflamed state.

BABY STEPS TO THE ELEVATOR!

There's a 90's movie called "What About Bob?" Bill Murray's character has some social anxieties and a phobia of elevators. His psychotherapist encourages him to just take "baby steps to the elevator." While I'm not a psychotherapist, my encouragement to start this program is the same. Do the one-week 7-Day Reset and go "all in," and then work on modifying your lifestyle for the long haul. Maybe start with getting meals, pressed juices, or quick snacks prepped through lunch, and then the second half of the day is more relaxed while you work on modifying your habits. Trust me, your body will thank you by craving the right foods at the right times. Before long, your circadian rhythms will be on track and driving you!

You can start turning the diet into a lifestyle for you and your family by making small changes every week. You can do it with a little planning. First, get in the habit of keeping snacks with you. Preparing meals and snacks for your family takes little time, but it can make all the difference in their health. Americans are the sickest nation in the world, and it's because of the way we eat. According to the CDC, nearly one out of five children or adolescents is obese. If your family is overweight, it's your duty as a parent to do better.

Start with small shifts in behaviors. Stop eating white foods (complex carbs) at breakfast today. Next week stop eating white foods at lunch. The green drink at lunch is key; our body feels full when we have enough nutrients. Stop eating dinner after 8 p.m., preferably 7 p.m. This is another huge game changer for people. I see entire families walking around with obvious signs of metabolic syndrome, like big bellies, double chins, and round chubby faces. You simply can't eat at night; it's a killer.

If you start eating nuts or fruits at breakfast and greens at lunch, you'll find that you can eat cooked vegetables and foods from the white group (complex carbs) at dinner and still lose weight. If you are going to eat red meat at dinner after 6 p.m., save it for Friday. You will be amazed at how your digestion improves.

I used to eat salads at night for dinner because I thought it would keep me from gaining weight. I could never fall asleep before midnight; I had no idea the dinner salad gave my body too much kinetic energy to fall asleep at a normal hour. Now I fall asleep by 10:30-11 p.m. and wake up at 6:30 a.m. without an alarm; it's incredible how much better I feel in the morning, and I don't need to set three alarms anymore!

More people are working remotely than ever, which makes following this program even easier. Do some meal prepping a couple of evenings per week so you can reach into the fridge for a snack or pop something into the oven to cook while you work.

I'm now over two years into the 7X Method and I look better than I did 20 years ago! I get comments that I look as if I work out a lot, and I don't. The only thing I changed was my diet. It's so profound I had to bring it to this country and write a book about it.

Here is another way to roll out the 7X Method:

- Week 1: Stop eating foods from the white group at breakfast and only drink coffee between 7 and 9 a.m. instead of all day long. Start eating nuts, berries, and fruits before noon. If you are one of those people who says, "I just like one small piece of dark chocolate after dinner," . . . you know who you are! 7-9 a.m. is the time to eat your chocolate.

- Week 2: Stop eating foods from the white group at lunchtime. Have a green drink and some green veggies or salad for lunch. Add some protein to stay full if you need to.

- Week 3: Start incorporating a late afternoon (3-5 a.m.) snack of non-green veggies, juice, or tropical fruit like pineapple, papaya, or mango.

- Week 4: Make it a goal to have either herbal tea, kombucha, or a small serving of beans, lentils, or other legumes (like a spoonful of peanut butter) between 5 and 6 p.m.

- Week 5: The idea is that you're eating so frequently throughout the day and keeping your blood sugar levels even, so you don't need to stuff yourself at night. You can still have your usual dinner with your family consisting of animal protein, food from the white group, and some cooked vegetables. Just try to make it a smaller portion, so you're not eating your biggest meal at night and sitting around. Instead of watching television after dinner, do one chore that requires standing and being active. Vacuum or do laundry. The bonus is that your days off on the weekend will actually be days off and not chore days.

If you do not work from home or you work a job where you cannot control the time of your meal breaks, but you can drink whenever/whatever you want, here is an alternate version of the 7X Method. The idea is to keep stable blood sugar levels throughout the day and get the desired electric charges from food to recalibrate your metabolism.

LIQUID-BASED PLAN (See also "The 7-Day Reset" pg 78)

- 7-9 a.m.: Coffee or tea, nut/berry smoothie

- 10 a.m.: One piece of fruit or natural fruit juice (no mainstream brand or other pasteurized juices)

- 1 p.m.: Green drink/smoothie and salad with protein; red meat is good

- 4 p.m.: Carrot/ginger juice, V8, or you can drink a hot soup

- 5 p.m.: Kombucha, herbal tea, or a spoonful of peanut butter or hummus

- 6 p.m.: Dinner with family consists of a small serving from the white foods group, cooked green or non-green vegetables (raw veggies have too much energy), light protein like fish or poultry (no red meat at dinner)

Eating this diet for seven days will cause a noticeable shift in cognition, but if you stay with it for three months or more, you will have mental clarity that you haven't felt in years, if ever. You may have a spiritual awakening or be aware of things you never noticed before. Some old patterns and addictions may finally subside. Sleep quality improves. You may tolerate stressful events better because your entire being is functioning at a higher frequency. Who hasn't wished for more patience with their kids? When your body is more coherent electrically, you are more in tune with your spirit, soul, and body.

Working six years in the American hospital system motivated me to learn how to use food as medicine. My dream is to get hospitals on board with this eating program and stop feeding our sick people food that looks like it's one step up from jail food. My goal is to reach millions of people and teach them to help themselves. I want my readers to improve their health by eating the right foods at the right time and by sharing the information with their friends and family. I want to create a community of elevated consciousness.

CHAPTER
9

Meal Planning
and Recipes

This first menu for the 7-Day Reset was designed for variety. Some people cannot eat the same food two days in a row. Some people can have the same berry smoothie for breakfast and green drink every day for lunch and be perfectly happy so I created the streamlined version. The streamlined version is listed after the variety version. You may have food sensitivities that you need to avoid. For example, hummus and lentils give me bloat and water retention for days, so I choose to have herbal tea or kombucha for the orange group. For the yellow group, I often grab a piece of dried mango or a carrot juice. It also depends on your appetite. Men usually need to eat more than women.

Here's a quiz that will help you determine which version of the 7-Day Reset that you want to do, variety or streamlined? Score yourself 1 point for "True" and 2 points for "False."

1. When I take home leftovers from a restaurant, they usually sit in my fridge until I throw them out.

    ☐ True
    ☐ False

2. I can't eat the same thing 2 days in a row.

    ☐ True
    ☐ False

3. I don't mind spending 45-60 minutes or more per day in the kitchen to follow recipes

    ☐ True
    ☐ False

4. I like experimenting with foods from different cuisines

    ☐ True
    ☐ False

5. In the past, I have felt very unsatisfied drinking juices, smoothies, or meal replacement shakes when trying to lose weight; it's definitely not something I could stick with long-term.

    ☐ True
    ☐ False

6. I work from home and have the flexibility to eat when I want. My job allows me to take meal breaks when I need to eat.

   ☐ True
   ☐ False

7. I don't easily feel overwhelmed when I learn complex concepts

   ☐ True
   ☐ False

8. I get excited about making big changes! People describe me as being someone who "jumps right in"

   ☐ True
   ☐ False

9. I take pride in paying attention to small details.

   ☐ True
   ☐ False

10. I usually plan my meals once a week and shop based on my meal plan.

    ☐ True
    ☐ False

Add your total score with True = 1 point and False = 2 points. If you score between 10 and 12, you will likely adhere to the Variety Version of the 7-Day Reset and you can find your plan following this paragraph. If you scored between 13 and 20, you will likely prefer the Streamlined Version of the 7-Day Reset. You can find this version of the 7-Day Reset following the variety version. You can also combine the two versions according to your taste; this is what I have done long-term. Some days I am really busy and I have to do the streamlined version. Some days I am really hungry and I want to do more of the Variety version.

SAMPLE MEAL PLAN–HIGH VARIETY VERSION

Here is a sample of the diet for those who like variety. Choose the foods you like from the list and insert them at the appropriate time of day. Remember, the biggest priority is to eat the right type of food at the right time of day, not necessarily to follow this meal plan exactly. It's a lot of food. You don't have to eat all seven groups every day. I gave you seven options so you have examples of things you can eat when you are hungry. If it's 2:30 in the afternoon and you are just having lunch, look at the clock. It's ideal to have a steak skewer from the red group and since you are almost to the yellow group, you can also have a non-green veggie like a baked sweet potato. If you are eating dinner at 5:30 p.m., have something from the orange group and the white group.

Try not to skip one of the food groups seven days in a row. For example, it can be hard for me to eat fruit between 9-11 a.m., but I can sip on a pressed juice. Usually, I only drink half the bottle and save the rest for the next day; this helps save money and also keeps me from eating too much. I also had a hard time with the orange group but I can drink an herbal tea or kombucha at this time while I prep dinner. Or if I am starving before dinner, I can swallow a spoonful of peanut butter to calm the hangry.

DAY 1:

7 - 9 a.m.

- Coffee/tea with nut milk (If desired)

- Purple smoothie - made in a blender

- 8 ounces coconut water

- 1/4 cup blueberries or blackberries

- 1/4 cup cranberries or dragon fruit or other dark fruit, e.g., plums, figs, prunes

- 1/4 of a lemon

- Add 1 date only if extremely sour

- Mix and enjoy

9–11 a.m.

- Apple or orange

11–1 p.m.

- Green drink

- 1 green apple

- 1/4 cup cilantro

- 1/4 parsley

- 1 cup cucumber

- 1 cup fresh mint leaves (or kale, depends on what is available at the store)

- Small wedge of lemon

- Coconut water

- If you live in a colder climate and you prefer something warm for lunch, an alternative is to have balsamic shaved brussels sprouts instead of a salad. Alternatively, at 1 p.m. you can have your salad with protein on it.

1–3 p.m.

- 2 hardboiled or deviled eggs, 6 oz fish, nitrate-free sliced turkey, or seasoned chicken breast

3–5 p.m.

- Snap peas/pea pods or carrot sticks. You can have these with the hummus if it's closer to 5:00 p.m.

5–6 p.m.

- Lentil soup or hummus

6–7 p.m.

- Oven-roasted potatoes with herbs and olive oil

- Rotisserie chicken (if desired, depends on appetite)

DAY 2

7–9 a.m.

- Coffee or tea if desired

- Strawberry-banana smoothie, mix in blender:

- Strawberries

- 1 banana

- Tart cherry, pomegranate, or REAL cranberry (not sugar cocktail) juice or coconut water or canned light coconut milk

9–11 a.m.

- ½-1 whole grapefruit, depending on size and appetite

11–1 p.m.

- Green drink:

- 1 apple

- ¼ cup Italian flat leaf parsley

- ¼ cup mint

- ¼ cup spinach, kale, or watercress

- Lemon or lime

- 1 date if sweetness is needed

- Mixed greens Salad: dressing made of coconut oil, apple cider vinegar or lemon and herbs, nothing creamy

-or-

- Zucchini "spaghetti" noodles with vegan pesto

1–3 p.m.

- One 6-ounce piece of salmon pan fried in olive oil with skin on or baked

3–5 p.m.

- Baked butternut squash blended with bone broth and tarragon

5–6 p.m.

- 2 ounces hummus with carrots, celery, and yellow pepper strips or aromatic tea if no appetite

6–7 p.m.

- ½ cup raw oatmeal, add cinnamon, 1 tsp honey and half an apple if desired

DAY 3

7–9 a.m.

- Coffee or tea

- Raw cacao chocolate mousse and fresh berries

- (Or berry smoothie)

9–11 a.m.

- 1 piece of fruit

- Hot water with squeezed lemon and honey

11–1 p.m.

- Green drink (and/or salad, no nuts, no tomatoes, or fruits unless they are green)

- Kale

- Watercress

- Cilantro

- Parsley

- Lemon

- Apple

- 1 date or stevia

- Himalayan salt

- Coconut water

- Broccoli soup

1–3 p.m.

- Grilled chicken breast or 3-6 oz of other protein

3–5 p.m.

- Sliced avocado and tomato with homemade dressing: olive oil, balsamic, and basil

- Or oven-roasted root vegetables, warmed veggies are nice in cold climates

5–6 p.m.

- Cannellini bean soup

6–7 p.m.

- 1 cup of brown rice with *Bragg* or coconut aminos, gluten-free tamari or nutritional yeast

- If you feel really hungry, add some cooked vegetables like bok choy, snap peas, bamboo shoots, water chestnuts and/or a little protein like shrimp or cod

DAY 4

7–9 a.m.

- Coffee with 1 tbsp coconut or MCT oil, some people like to add collagen powder to their coffee

- Blackberry smoothie

9–11 a.m.

- Fruit salad

11–1 p.m.

- Green drink and large mixed greens salad or

- Green veggie cakes

1–3 p.m.

- 6 oz burger no bun: turkey, beef, or buffalo

3–5 p.m.

- Papaya, avocado, or other non-green vegetables like carrot sticks and peanut butter

5–6 p.m.

- Yellow lentil dahl or lentil soup

6–7 p.m.

- Roasted cauliflower, add chicken, grilled shrimp, or seafood on the side if you like more protein

DAY 5

7–9 a.m.

- Coffee or tea

- Blackberry smoothie

9–11 a.m.

- Cantaloupe, watermelon, honeydew melon

11–1 p.m.

- Mixed greens salad -or-

- Grilled asparagus

- Green drink, wheatgrass or spirulina mixed in water

1–3 p.m.

- Lamb in mint sauce (apple cider vinegar or fresh lemon juice, mint leaves, salt)

3–5 p.m.

- Fresh carrot juice or sliced avocado with lemon and olive oil -or-

- Baked root vegetables (Yes, at 3 p.m. you can have a nice platter of lamb and oven-roasted root vegetables)

5–6 p.m.

- 2 tbsp hummus with carrot sticks and celery or aromatic tea, depending on your appetite

6–7 p.m.

- Gluten-free pasta with vegan pesto sauce, toss in broiled shrimp if you would like more protein

DAY 6

7–9 a.m.

- Coffee or tea, 1 serving dark chocolate

- Berry smoothie

9–11 a.m.

- Fresh fruit

11–1 p.m.

- Green drink: coconut water, kiwi, spirulina, algae, chlorella

- Salad, may layer on eggs, fish, or chicken if you need more protein or

- Steamed spinach

1–3 p.m.

- 6 oz salmon or other protein

3–5 p.m.

- Mango smoothie: frozen mangos, coconut water, cardamon spice if desired

5–6 p.m.

- Mint tea, lentil soup or hummus

6–8 p.m.

- Oatmeal with cinnamon and honey -or-

- Gluten-free pancakes or waffles with eggs

DAY 7

7–9 a.m.

- Coffee or tea and homemade chocolate mousse

- Berry smoothie

9–11 a.m.

- ½ grapefruit or other water bearing fruit such as pineapple

11–1 p.m.

- Green drink and

- Mixed greens salad -or-

- Green tomatillo soup

1–3 p.m.

- Kimchee chicken and bok choy

3–5 p.m.

- Papaya or mango -or-

- White fish dip with carrots and celery

5–6 p.m.

- Chamomile tea

6–7 p.m.

- Quinoa with fish

HIGH VARIETY VERSION CHART

If you look at this chart, there are a variety of items from each colored food group.

TIME	MON	TUES	WED	THUR	FRI	SAT	SUN
PURPLE 7 a.m.–9 a.m. -Electro-Pulsating, Start-up Energy	Coffee or tea w/nut milk blueberry smoothie	Coffee or tea w/nut milk straw-berry smooth-ie	Coffee/ tea w/nut milk blueber-ry smoothie or cacao mousse	Coffee w/ MCT oil black-ber-ry smoothie	Coffee/ tea w/nut milk blueber-ry smoothie	Coffee/ tea w/nut milk, choco-late, berry smoothie	Coffee/ tea choco-late mouse or berry smooth-ie
BLUE 9 a.m.–11 a.m. -Electro-Lu-minous, Light Energy	Apple or orange	grape-fruit	pear	Fruit salad	Canta-loupe wa-ter-mel-on, or Honey-dew melon	Fresh fruit	Grape-fruit pineap-ple or other fresh fruit

GREEN **11–1 p.m.** Electro-Kinetic Energy	Green drink & salad or shaved brussels sprouts	Green drink & salad or zucchini noodles w pesto	Green drink & salad or broccoli soup	Green drink & salad or green veggie cakes	Green drink & salad or grilled asparagus	Green drink & salad or steamed spinach	Green drink & salad or tomatillo soup
RED **1–3 p.m.** Electro-Thermic Energy	2 eggs or 6 oz fish or 6 oz chicken/ turkey	6 oz salmon pan fried with skin on	6 oz grilled steak or chicken breast	6 oz burger: beef, turkey, or bison	Lamb in mint sauce	6 oz salmon or other protein	Kimchee chicken and bok choy
YELLOW **3–5 p.m.** Electro-Static Energy	Snap peas carrot sticks	Butternut squash soup with tarragon	Sliced avocado and tomato w balsamic	Avocado or celery and peanut butter	Oven roasted root vegetables	Mango smoothie with cardamon	Papaya or white fish dip with celery and carrots
ORANGE **5–6 p.m.** Electro-Magnetic Energy	Lentil soup or hummus	2 oz hummus celery carrots peppers	Cannellini bean soup or peanut butter	Yellow lentil dahl	Hummus celery carrots peppers	Mint tea lentil soup or hummus	Chamomile tea
WHITE **6 - 7 p.m.** Electro-Insular Energy, Inward	Oven-roasted potatoes w/herbs, rotisserie chicken if hungry	Oatmeal with apple and honey	1 cup of rice with aminos, add veggies or shrimp to make a stir fry	Roasted cauliflower, grilled chicken or seafood	Gluten free pasta with vegan pesto, add shrimp if needed	Gluten free pancakes or waffles with eggs	Baked fish and quinoa

GROCERY LIST FOR 7-DAY RESET HIGH VARIETY VERSION (ORGANIC, NON-GMO ONLY)

- Organic coffee or black tea (if desired)

- Herbal/aromatic tea (for 5-6 p.m.)

- Nut milk for coffee or tea

- Canned light coconut milk x4 for smoothies (7-9 a.m.) or coconut rice

- Bananas for smoothies

- Blueberries, blackberries, strawberries, raspberries, cherries, fresh or frozen (I pick 3 bags of frozen berries per week for breakfast smoothies)

- Mixed greens for salads if desired, I prefer to make green drinks with avocado for my lunch

- Dates for sweetening smoothies and making the chocolate mousse for breakfast

- Tart cherry, pomegranate, or REAL cranberry (not sugar cocktail) juice if you can't have coconut for smoothies

- Coconut water

- Almonds, 2 cups unsalted

- Oranges or grapefruits

- Kiwi or pear, if available for green drink or to eat as a snack

- Green apples

- Lemons

- Limes

- Cranberries, dragon fruit, or acai from freezer section for breakfast smoothies

- Cucumbers, 1-2 for crudité or green drinks

- Celery, 1 bunch is enough for crudité and lentil soup

- Carrots

- Yellow peppers for crudité if desired

- Cilantro

- Italian flat leaf parsley

- Mint

- Spirulina and chlorella, often you can get these both in a powdered drink mix

- Kale

- Spinach

- Watercress greens

- Broccoli for soup or pre-made broccoli soup

- 1 russet baking potato

- Chicken breasts

- Nitrate-free sliced turkey

- Shrimp, fresh or frozen, peeled, and de-veined, enough to add to dinner if you are hungry

- Lamb chops, 6 oz

- Fresh cold-water fish for grilling, 3-6 oz fillets, Coho or Sockeye are great, avoid "Atlantic" salmon

- Whitefish dip, nitrate free for snacking with crudité between 2-5 p.m. if desired

- Buffalo, beef, or turkey burger

- Eggs

- Bone broth, 2 quarts chicken

- Fresh ginger root, for lentil soup

- Fresh turmeric root, for lentil soup

- Fresh or frozen watermelon for mid-morning snack

- Mango, fresh or frozen for mid-morning or late-afternoon snack

- Papaya, fresh or frozen for mid-morning or late-afternoon snack

- Garlic, 1 head

- Carrot sticks for lentil soup and crudité

- Snap pea pods for crudité or stir fry

- Onions for lentil soup and tomatillo soup

- Hummus pre-made or chickpeas and tahini to make from scratch

- Olive oil

- Gluten-free tamari

- *Bragg* or coconut amino acids

- Coconut oil

- Bok choy, oven-roasted side dish or stir fry, I like baby bok choy the best

- Water chestnuts for stir fry

- Bamboo shoots

- Apple cider vinegar

- Avocados, 2 bags for smoothies

- Baking soda, aluminum-free, for soaking produce

- Fresh or frozen squash for soup

- Zucchini noodles for lunch

- Asparagus for lunch, you can wrap in turkey bacon

- Green veggie cakes, frozen

- Brussels sprouts

- Balsamic glaze

- Frozen or fresh root vegetables for oven roasting

- Cocoa powder for chocolate mousse or 85% cacao chocolate bar for breakfast

- Gluten-free pancake or waffle mix

- Honey, stevia, dates, or monk fruit for sweetening if you need to wean your sweet tooth

- Raw oatmeal, avoid instant if possible

- 3X 15oz cans of cannellini beans or 1 bag of lentils, depending on which soup you want

- Gluten-free pasta

- Vegan pesto sauce or 1 bunch basil, raw cashews and 1 bag pine nuts

The streamlined version is a simpler plan with less variety for those who find this easier to implement.

- **7–9 a.m.**–Coffee or tea, real dark chocolate (optional) nut/berry smoothie (optional)

- **10 a.m.–**1 piece of fruit or real fruit juice (no mainstream brands or other pasteurized juices)

- **12/1 p.m.–**Green drink/smoothie and salad with protein, red meat is ok

- **4 p.m.**–carrot/ginger juice, V8, or you can drink a hot soup

- **5 p.m.**–Kombucha, herbal tea, or a spoonful of peanut butter or hummus

- **6 p.m.–**Dinner consists of a small serving from the white foods group, green or non-green cooked vegetables (raw veggies have too much energy), light protein like fish or poultry, no red meat at dinner except on Friday

🔥 **HOT TIP**

If you are too busy working to meal prep juice, this site has a 20 pack available, or find a local juice shop to make things easier: Juicefromtheraw.com, pick seven green juices to drink between 11 a.m. and 2 p.m., and order seven of the "Immunity Boost" with carrot juice to drink 3-5 p.m. For the 10 a.m. slot, you can buy a combination of the shots and any fruit juice that looks good to you. I prefer the shots because it's less sugar overall (you only need a small dose to get the nutrients your body needs).

I recently tried juices from **PureGreen.com** and loved that they had less sugar (apple juice is a cheap filler). "Golden Girl" is great for the 3-5 p.m. time slot because it's made of turmeric, carrot, pineapple, lemon, and ginger. Some other options are Squeezed.com, Pressed.com, Rawfountainjuice.com, Rawjuicery.com, Cleanjuice.com. The list is endless. I suggest doing an online search and also search for coupons.

If you are too busy to cook, you can order custom meals from an organic meal delivery service near you.

- Lunch=red meat or any variety of protein and green veggies no carbs

- Dinner=plant-based protein, fish or poultry, veggies, and a carb

MONDAY, DAY 1

7–9 a.m. (If desired, you may skip this meal and opt for exercise outdoors in sunlight if your schedule permits.)

- Coffee or tea, you may add nut milk

- Dark chocolate (optional)

- Berry smoothie (optional) depends on your appetite and weight loss goals, you can add this later in your diet to maintain your weight

Blackberry Breakfast Smoothie

- Soak 1 cup of raw almonds in water overnight if possible, or at least 10 minutes (soaking almonds helps make the nutrients more absorbable)

- 32 oz pressed coconut water, this brand is the best tasting for smoothies, you can substitute a can of light coconut milk if you can't find this, just add 1 can of water also

- 1 bag of frozen organic blackberries

- Juice of 1 lemon or lime (optional)

- Himalayan salt

- 2 dates or honey (optional, try to wean yourself of the sweet tooth)

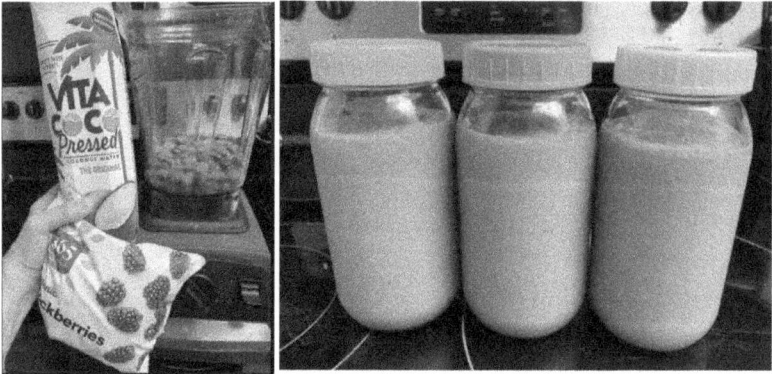

9–11 a.m.

- 1 piece of fruit or a real fruit juice

12–2 p.m.

- Green drink/juice

- Salad with a protein added, fruits and veggies optional, (no nuts, dairy/cheese/ranch dressing, gluten/croutons), vinaigrette dressing or olive oil with balsamic or lemon juice

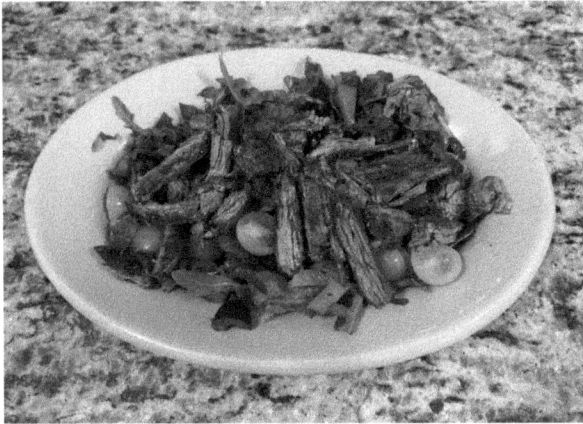

Cucumber Avocado Green Smoothie (or grab any green cold-pressed juice from the store)

- 1 L coconut water

- Cucumber, I prefer the English kind

- Watercress

- Dandelion greens

- Cilantro

- Parsley

- 2 small avocados

- Juice of 1 lime

- Himalayan salt, dash of olive oil

- If the veggie taste is too blah for you, you can use honey or dates to sweeten or another fruit, like kiwi. You can also go the other direction and add jalapeño and extra cilantro.

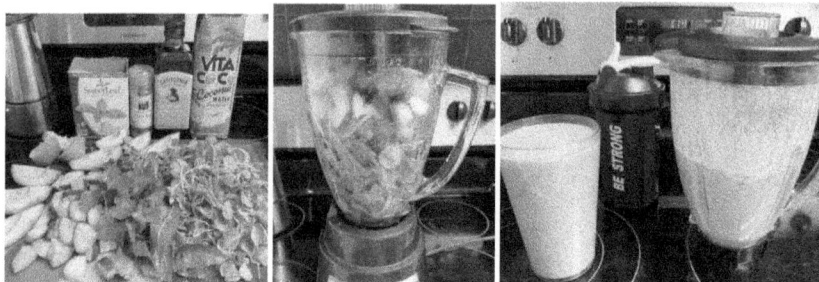

3–5 p.m.

- Carrot or other veggie juice

5–6 p.m.

- Kombucha or herbal tea or spoonful of hummus or peanut butter

6–7 p.m.

- Mojo Mahi-Mahi (or other white fish), veggies, and citrus-cilantro rice (Feeds two people.)

- Pre-heat oven to 400°

- Juice 2 oranges, 1 lemon, and 1 lime and put in blender with 4 garlic cloves, ½ an onion, 1 tsp oregano, 1 tsp cumin,

½ tsp salt, ½ tsp pepper, and 2 TBSP olive oil. Blend. This is enough marinade for a whole family, or it makes leftovers if you're only feeding 2 people.

- Marinate 1 pound of white fish for 20 minutes in a glass baking dish, this marinade is also great with steak for 2-3 hours, or with chicken for 1 day

- Sauté 1 cup of rice in 1 tbsp of coconut oil until toasted

- Add 2 cups of chicken bone broth, 1 tbsp orange rind, ¼ cup fresh cilantro (or 2 tbsp dried cilantro), and 2 tbsp mojo sauce

- Boil & reduce to simmer until cooked thoroughly

- Bake fish in the oven for approximately 15 minutes depending on the thickness of your filet; a good rule of thumb is about 6 minutes for each ½ inch

- Prepare your steamed veggies as directed

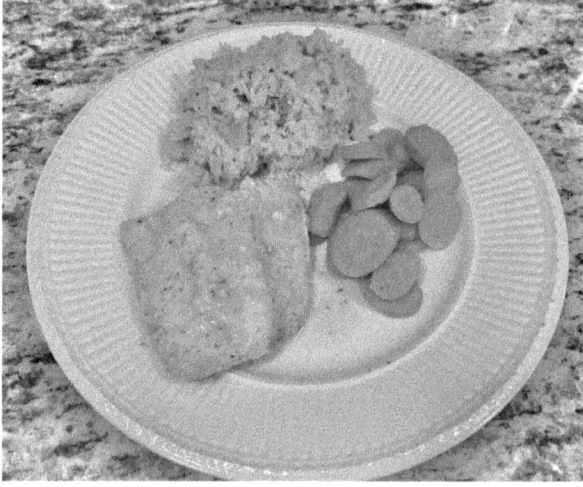

TUESDAY, DAY 2

7–9 a.m. (If desired, you may skip this meal and opt for exercise outdoors in sunlight if your schedule permits.)

- Coffee or tea, you may add nut milk

- Dark chocolate, 72% cacao or greater (optional)

- Berry smoothie (optional) depends on your appetite and weight loss goals, you can add this later in your diet to maintain your weight

9–11 a.m.

- 1 piece of fruit or REAL juice

12–2 p.m.

- Green drink/juice

- Salad with a protein added, fruits and veggies optional, (no nuts, dairy/cheese/ranch dressing, gluten/croutons), vinaigrette dressing

3–5 p.m.

- Carrot or other veggie juice like V8

5–6 p.m.

- Kombucha or herbal tea or spoonful of hummus or peanut butter

6–7 p.m.

Veggie Stir Fry (Feeds two people.)

- Pick three vegetables: snow pea pods, carrots, mushrooms, broccoli, bok choy, bamboo shoots, water chestnuts

- Pick a protein like ½ pound of shrimp or 2 chicken breasts, or 4 chicken thighs

Sauté together until the garlic is cooked, stir often, don't burn:

- 2 garlic cloves

- 1 tbsp ginger fresh or 1 tsp ginger powder

- 1 tbsp coconut oil

- Add the veggies and cook until they are al dente (no soggy veggies please) and set aside

- Add in your protein and sauté until they're cooked thoroughly

- Mix together ¼ cup water, ¼ cup tamari or soy sauce, and 1 tbsp cornstarch, then add to the proteins cooking in the pan, this should make a sauce

- Add the veggies back in and remove the pan from heat

- Serve with 1 cup of rice maximum, <1 cup if trying to lose weight. I like the sauce from the stir fry on my rice but that may not be enough flavor for your taste buds. You may season additionally with *Bragg* or coconut aminos, gluten-free tamari, or nutritional yeast.

WEDNESDAY, DAY 3

7–9 a.m. (If desired, you may skip this meal and opt for exercise in sunlight if your schedule permits.)

- Coffee or tea, you may add nut milk

- Dark chocolate (optional)

- Berry smoothie (optional) depends on your appetite and weight loss goals, you can add this later in your diet to maintain your weight

9–11 a.m.

- 1 piece of fruit or REAL juice

12–2 p.m.

- Green drink/juice

- Salad with a protein added, fruits and veggies optional, (no nuts, dairy/cheese/ranch dressing, gluten/croutons), vinaigrette dressing

3–5 p.m.

- Carrot or other veggie juice like V8

5–6 p.m.

- Kombucha or herbal tea or spoonful of hummus or peanut butter

6–7 p.m.

Chicken Fajitas (Feeds two people.)

- Cut 1 pound of chicken breast into bite-size pieces

- In a skillet, heat 1 tbsp coconut or avocado oil with

- 1 tsp cumin

- 1 tsp paprika

- ½ tsp garlic powder or 2 cloves garlic

- ½ tsp oregano

- ½ tsp black pepper

- ¼ tsp cayenne (optional, may need more or less depending on your preference)

- ½ tsp Himalayan salt

- *Alternatively, you may use a pre-mixed sauce to save time, watch for preservatives*

- Add diced chicken and sauté until meat is firm

- Add 1 sliced bell pepper and 1 sliced onion

- Mix together ¼ cup of water, juice of 1 lime, and 1 tbsp cornstarch and stir into sauce to thicken, then remove from heat

- Serve with gluten-free tortillas, pico de gallo, and guacamole

- Optional: plantain chips to dip the extra guac and pico

THURSDAY, DAY 4

7–9 a.m. (If desired, you may skip this meal and opt for exercise outdoors in sunlight if your schedule permits.)

- Coffee or tea, you may add nut milk

- Dark chocolate (optional)

- Berry smoothie (optional) depends on your appetite and weight loss goals, you can add this later in your diet to maintain your weight

Raspberry Lime Breakfast Smoothie

- Soak 1 cup of almonds at least 1 hour

- 1 can light coconut milk and 32 oz coconut water or 32 oz pressed coconut water

- 1 bag frozen organic raspberries

- Juice of 1 lime or lemon (this helps preserve it in your fridge for a couple days, you will get three servings)

- Himalayan salt

- 2 dates or honey (If you need the sweetness, try to do without)

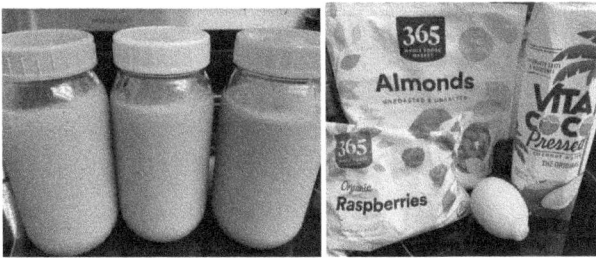

9–11 a.m.

- 1 piece of fruit or REAL juice

12–2 p.m.

- Green drink/juice

- Salad with a protein added, fruits and veggies optional, (no nuts, dairy/cheese/ranch dressing, gluten/croutons), vinaigrette dressing

My Favorite Green Smoothie

- 1 L coconut water (the coconut water is actually better at this time period than the pressed coconut which is better suited for the 7-9 a.m. electric charge, shown here in the photo)

- ½ bag frozen passion fruit

- Watercress

- Dandelion greens (dandelion leaf is known as a potassium-sparing diuretic, meaning it is high in potassium and works to reduce water retention and bloating)

- Swiss chard

- 2 small avocados or 1 medium avocado

- Juice of 1 lime

- Himalayan salt, a dash of olive oil

- Honey or dates (optional)

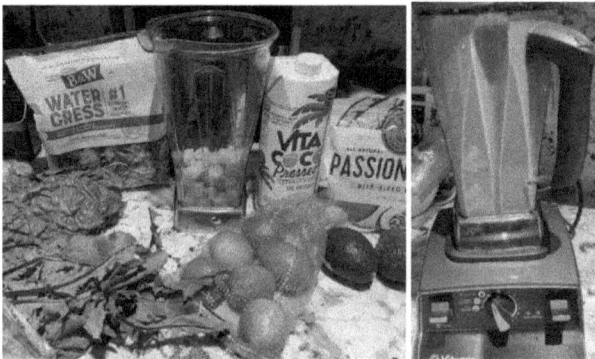

3–5 p.m.

- Carrot or other veggie juice like V8

5–6 p.m.

- Kombucha or herbal tea or spoonful of hummus or peanut butter

6–7 p.m.

Sweet and Sour Chicken (Or use shrimp. Pair with coconut basmati rice. Feeds two people.)

- Prepare basmati rice as directed on the package, substitute 1 can of light coconut milk and chicken bone broth for water (roughly 1 cup of dry rice to 1 ½ -2 cups of liquid).

- Dice 1 pound of chicken breast or thighs and marinate in 1 tbsp gluten-free tamari or soy sauce.

- Prepare sweet and sour sauce.

- Combine in a saucepan and bring to a boil.

- 1 can of crushed pineapple with juice, 2 tbsp siracha or more depending on your preference, 2 tbsp tamari/soy/ fish sauce, 2 tbsp vinegar, or 2 tbsp lime juice.

- Stir in 1 tbsp cornstarch with ¼ cup water (premixed) to thicken the sauce and remove from heat

- Chop 2 garlic cloves, 1 carrot, 1 celery stalk, and ½ onion, and sauté in a large pan with 1 tbsp coconut oil.

- Add 1 can of bamboo shoots and diced chicken and cook thoroughly.

- Add sweet and sour pineapple sauce to chicken and vegetable mixture and serve over rice.

FRIDAY, DAY 5

7–9 a.m. (If desired, you may skip this meal and opt for exercise in sunlight if your schedule permits.)

- Coffee or tea, you may add nut milk

- Dark chocolate (optional)

- Berry smoothie (optional) depends on your appetite and weight loss goals, you can add this later in your diet to maintain your weight

9–11 a.m.

- 1 piece of fruit or REAL juice

12–2 p.m.

- Green drink/juice

- Salad with a protein added, fruits and veggies optional, (no nuts, dairy/cheese/ranch dressing, gluten/croutons), vinaigrette dressing

3–5 p.m.

- Carrot or other veggie juice like V8

5–6 p.m.

- Kombucha or herbal tea or spoonful of hummus or peanut butter

6–7 p.m.

Chimichurri Steak with Grilled Veggies and Potatoes (Feeds two people.)

- Dice together 1 russet potato (optional if your grocery store doesn't have plantains or yucca), 1 yellow squash, and 1 zucchini. Toss with 1 tbsp olive oil, salt, and pepper. Either grill with your steaks, sauté with 1 tbsp olive oil, or oven roast at 400° for 30 minutes.

- Chimichurri sauce, pulse the following ingredients in a food processor or blender:

- 1 cup parsley, 1 cup cilantro, ½ cup olive oil, 2 garlic cloves, ¼ cup apple cider vinegar or lemon juice, ½-1 tsp salt, ½ tsp black pepper, and red pepper flakes to taste. There will be plenty leftover which is great for seafood marinades as well.

- Slice sweet or green plantains and sauté in coconut oil.

- Grill or sauté 2 churrasco steaks to your temperature preference. I prefer bison over beef but either is fine as long as it's grass-fed.

- Top steaks with chimichurri sauce.

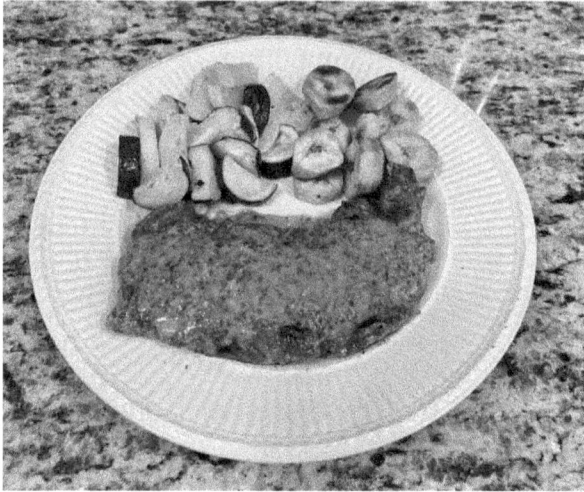

SATURDAY, DAY 6

7–9 a.m. (If desired, you may skip this meal and opt for exercise in sunlight if your schedule permits.)

- Coffee or tea, you may add nut milk

- Dark chocolate (optional)

- Berry smoothie (optional) depends on your appetite and weight loss goals, you can add this later in your diet to maintain your weight

9–11 a.m.

- 1 piece of fruit or REAL juice

12–2 p.m.

- Green drink/juice

- Salad with a protein added, fruits and veggies optional, (no nuts, dairy/cheese/ranch dressing, gluten/croutons), vinaigrette dressing or balsamic glaze

3–5 p.m.

- Carrot or other veggie juice like V8

5–6 p.m.

- Kombucha or herbal tea or spoonful of hummus or peanut butter

6–7 p.m.

- Oven-roasted potatoes with herbs, baked chicken, steamed veggies

- Marinate your chicken breasts or thighs 24 hours or more in Italian dressing or mojo sauce. Place in a glass baking dish.

- Preheat oven to 400°

- Wash your organic potatoes and dice them into 1" cubes.

- Toss potatoes with olive oil, fresh dill or parsley, Himalayan salt, and fresh ground black pepper (dried herbs and garlic powder are good too).

- Place on a cookie sheet lined with parchment paper and bake for approximately 30 minutes.

- Bake chicken for 20-25 minutes until internal temperature is 165°.

- Steam or sauté your favorite veggies in olive, coconut, or avocado oil.

SUNDAY, DAY 7

7–9 a.m. (If desired, you may skip this meal and opt for exercise in sunlight if your schedule permits.)

- Coffee or tea, you may add nut milk

- Dark chocolate (optional)

- Berry smoothie (optional) depends on your appetite and weight loss goals, you can add this later in your diet to maintain your weight

9–11 a.m.

- 1 piece of fruit or REAL juice

12–2 p.m.

- Green drink/juice

- Salad with a protein added, red meat is good at this time, fruits, and veggies optional, (no nuts, dairy/cheese/ranch dressing, gluten/croutons), vinaigrette dressing

3–5 p.m.

- Carrot or other veggie juice like V8

5–6 p.m.

- Kombucha or herbal tea or spoonful of hummus or peanut butter

6–7 p.m.

Walnut-Crusted Salmon, Broccoli, Sweet Potatoes (Feeds two people.)

- Preheat oven to 425°.

- Scrub your sweet potatoes clean and bake until tender, approximately 45 minutes.

- Combine salmon topping in a bowl: 1 tsp lemon zest, 2/3 cup chopped walnuts, ½ tsp garlic powder, ½ tsp onion powder, ½ tsp chipotle powder, 1 tbsp Dijon mustard, 2 tbsp maple syrup, 1 tbsp olive oil, salt, and pepper.

- Line a baking sheet with parchment paper and place salmon filets skin side down.

- Coat the top of the salmon filets with the topping.

- Clean your broccoli and place in a steamer or pot with very little water, don't boil the nutrients out of your veggies.

- Put salmon in the oven 6 minutes for every ½-inch of thick thickness. So, a 1-inch-thick filet will be 12 minutes.

- Enjoy your potato with grass fed butter and cinnamon.

7-DAY RESET STREAMLINED VERSION CHART

Time	Mon	Tues	Wed	Thur	Fri	Sat	Sun
PURPLE 7–9 a.m. Electro Pulsating, Start-up Energy	Coffee or tea w/nut milk, berry smoothie	Coffee or tea w/nut milk, berry smoothie	Coffee or tea w/nut milk, berry smoothie	Coffee or tea w/nut milk, berry smoothie	Coffee or tea w/nut milk, berry smoothie	Coffee or tea w/nut milk, berry smoothie	Coffee or tea w/nut milk, berry smoothie
BLUE 9–11 a.m. Electroluminous, Light Energy	REAL fruit juice or a piece of fruit	REAL fruit juice or a piece of fruit	REAL fruit juice or a piece of fruit	REAL fruit juice or a piece of fruit	REAL fruit juice or a piece of fruit	REAL fruit juice or a piece of fruit	REAL fruit juice or a piece of fruit
GREEN 11 - 1 p.m. Electro kinetic Energy	Green drink & salad w/protein (red meat optional)	Green drink & salad w/protein (red meat optional)	Green drink & salad w/protein (red meat optional)	Green drink & salad w/protein (red meat optional)	Green drink & salad w/protein (red meat optional)	Green drink & salad w/protein (red meat optional)	Green drink & salad w/protein (red meat optional)
RED 1–3 p.m. Electro thermic Energy	Protein was eaten with salad or can be a separate snack here	Protein was eaten with salad or can be a separate snack here	Protein was eaten with salad or can be a separate snack here	Protein was eaten with salad or can be a separate snack here	Protein was eaten with salad or can be a separate snack here	Protein was eaten with salad or can be a separate snack here	Protein was eaten with salad or can be a separate snack here
YELLOW 3–5 p.m. Electro-static Energy	Carrot/ ginger juice, V8, or hot soup	Carrot/ ginger juice, V8, or hot soup	Carrot/ ginger juice, V8, or hot soup	Carrot/ ginger juice, V8, or hot soup	Carrot/ ginger juice, V8, or hot soup	Carrot / ginger juice, V8, or hot soup	Carrot/ ginger juice, V8, or hot soup

ORANGE 5–6 p.m. Electro-magnetic Energy	Kom-bucha, herbal tea or spoon-ful of peanut butter or hum-mus	Kom-bucha, herbal tea or spoon-ful of peanut butter	Kombu-cha, herb-al tea or spoonful of peanut butter or hummus	Kom-bucha, herbal tea or spoon-ful of peanut butter	Kom-bucha, herbal tea or spoon-ful of peanut butter or hummus	Kom-bucha, herbal tea or spoon-ful of peanut butter or hummus	Kom-bucha, herbal tea or spoon-ful of peanut butter or hummus
WHITE 6–7 p.m. Electro Insular Energy, Inward	Mojo sea-soned white fish, cilantro rice, veggies	Rice with aminos, green veggies and shrimp to make a stir fry	Chicken fajitas or tacos w/GF tortillas, plantain chips and guac	Sweet and sour shrimp or chick-en w/ pine-apple & (co-conut) basmati rice	Steak w/ chi-michurri, grilled veggies, Yucca or potatoes or plan-tains	Oven roasted pota-toes w/ herbs, mojo chicken, steamed veggies	Pecan-Crusted salmon, broccoli, sweet potatoes

GROCERY LIST FOR 7-DAY RESET STREAMLINED VERSION (MEALS FOR 1 PERSON)

- 6 chicken breasts (1 mojo Saturday, 1 fajita Wednesday, 4 lunches/salads)

- 1 lb shrimp (Tuesday stir-fry, sweet and sour Thursday)

- 1/2 lb steak (chimichurri Friday)

- 1/2 lb white fish (Mojo Monday)

- 1/2 lb wild caught salmon (Sunday)

- 2X 6 oz buffalo or grass-fed beef steaks for salads/lunches

- Potatoes: 1 Yukon gold, 1 red, 1 sweet

- 1 small zucchini (1/2 for Monday, 1/2 Friday)

- 1 yellow squash

- 1 small plantain

- 1 bunch parsley

- 1 bunch cilantro

- 4 limes

- 3 lemons

- 2 oranges

- 3 carrots

- Celery

- Broccoli (for stir fry and salmon)

- 1 onion (fajita and sweet and sour shrimp)

- 1 head garlic

- 1 bell pepper (for fajita and stir-fry)

- 2 bags of lettuce for salads

- Guacamole (optional)

- Gluten-free tortillas

- Plantain chips (optional)

- Basmati rice

- 1 can coconut milk for rice

- 1 can pineapple

- Gluten-free soy or tamari

- Siracha

- Balsamic glaze or other vinegar

- Dijon mustard

- Walnuts

- Chicken bone broth for rice

- Cornstarch for sauces

- Baking soda to soak produce

- Herbal / aromatic tea (for 5-6 p.m.)

- Veggies for salads: olives, roasted red peppers, sundried tomatoes, artichokes, capers, whatever you like to eat (no cheese, nuts, or croutons)

- Peanut butter/hummus/herbal tea for 5-6 p.m.

- Coffee or tea (coconut/almond/other nut milk optional)

- Order the juices online (or buy 7 pieces of fruit for 9-11 a.m., 1 bag of dried mango or papaya for 3-5 p.m., 3 L coconut water + 6 kiwis + 2 bags watercress + 3 med avocados + cucumber + other greens +dates/honey for 11-1 p.m. green drink)

TESTIMONIALS

Melinda - 42 years old, female, married with 3 kids, works long hours remotely.

What was the #1 goal you hoped to achieve, and did you achieve it?

Health, and yes, I am getting there, I feel like I am moving in the right direction for a change!

What did you like about the 7x Method?

This program is amazing! I have lost 7 pounds in only 1.5 weeks! I love how easy it is. There are great meal suggestions but due to my busy life and lack of desire to cook, I purchased easy to grab foods and ate them during the indicated times. I still eat the things I love, and my energy levels are at an all-time high. I am one to try to listen to my body, so now knowing which foods at what times of day are good for it, helps me to be even more in tune with myself. I plan to use this for the rest of my life. Thank you!

What did you dislike about the 7x Method? Too hard to follow? Too much meal prep?

Meals were not mandatory only suggested so it worked for me. I made 1-2 meals off the program, and they were delicious. I mostly used grab and go veggies, hummus, kombucha, salad mixes, and nuts.

What did you like about the technology? Combining a Facebook group and using the Healthie app?

This app has it all. I have learned so much about how important gut health is. Before starting this program, I would be backed up for weeks at a time [with constipation]. Now I am every other day and hope to continue to improve in that area. Tracking what is going on internally really let me see where issues are and where I need to focus most. Also, seeing everyday how you are doing helped motivate me to keep it up and keep improving.

Did you have any issues with the technology?

No, it's great.

Would you continue the 7x Method long term? Would you recommend the 7x Method to a friend?

Yes!

Brenda - 41 years old, female, mother of 2 girls ages 3 and 5, works as a teacher. Brenda had gestational diabetes and her doctors think that she was probably pre-diabetic prior to becoming pregnant but she was never officially diagnosed.

Brenda initially tried the 7-Day Reset in fall of 2021 but quit after the holidays and then admittedly ate terribly for 6 months . . . too much southern comfort food! Was suffering from massive hemorrhoids and bilateral carpal tunnel syndrome that required regular trips to the chiropractor.

Brenda was feeling so unwell that she was considering going to the hospital. While she was driving, she glanced down at the emergency brake and noticed a piece of paper sticking up with the 7-Day Reset printed out on it. She was like "Oh My God! Dr. Sarah's diet!"

I'll never forget the day, July 3, 2022. I quit drinking alcohol and started adhering to the diet religiously." Fast forward four months and Brenda has lost 20 pounds; the hemorrhoids are gone and so is the carpal tunnel. "I haven't seen my chiropractor in over two months, I know he's mad at me, but I don't need him anymore!

Brenda orders shakes to help with the morning (chocolate or fruit), orders green shakes for lunch, and other snacks to help her eat all the right groups. She uses an app that links to the apple watch that will remind her to eat every 2.5 hours. She is doing a fabulous job getting the 7 food groups in almost every day, and she does it while talking in front of a group of high school students every day and taking care of two little girls and a husband!

Eduardo - 27-year-old male who desired to lose belly fat. Had the luxury of a personal chef and was very compliant with the program. Said it's the best he's ever felt in his life. He worked out every day with a personal trainer. His results are amazing for 1 week! He was motivated to continue on. Here is his exit survey:

What was your #1 goal that you hoped to achieve, and did you achieve it?

Lose belly fat. Yes.

What did you like about the 7x Method?

I loved that the fruits I had at specific times of the morning and day really made me feel like I was processing them in my body how I have been made to. Unbelievable and exciting, I even quit coffee because of how much I enjoyed having tea with almond milk.

What did you dislike about the 7x Method? Too hard to follow? Too much meal prep?

Meal prep is easy when you sort it out three days at a time, so I loved that part. Had much more energy this week, not hard to follow at all.

What did you like about the technology? Combining a Facebook group and using the Healthie app?

The app was very easy to use. I loved everything about it.

Did you have any issues with the technology?

I didn't experience any issues.

Would you continue the 7x Method long term? Would you recommend to a friend?

I would absolutely do this long-term. I haven't really stopped with it since I started.

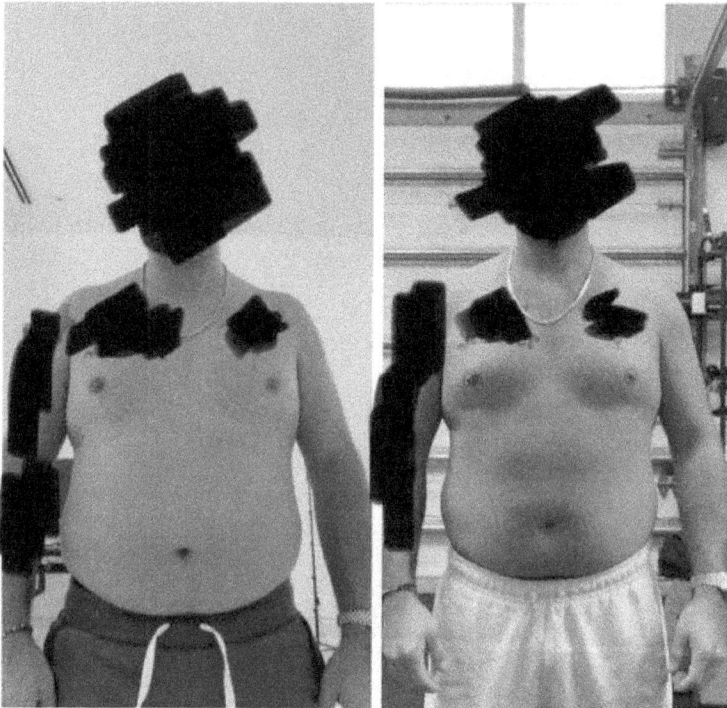

Kelly - 37-year-old female, 2 kids, youngest is 5. Can't fit into some of her pants or the waist is too tight on other pairs. Too much Christmas! Followed the diet 7 days and on the 8th day ate carbs at breakfast and was doubled over with stomach pain for hours. She realized that her digestion was much, much better on the diet, had no bloating and had more energy. Lost almost 1 pants size in the week. She said that eating 7 times per day was kind of annoying, but she was able to do it since she worked from home. Did not exercise while on the reset but wishes she would have so she would have gotten a bigger benefit. No photo submission.

Jillian - *I couldn't believe how easy this was to follow and I could still eat all the yummy foods I love! I had to get over "carb shaming" and make it okay to eat fruit and have carbs at night–which makes total sense! But in just less than a week, my digestion improved dramatically. My heartburn went away and I started having more energy. Could it really be this easy? I also lost ½ inch everywhere and I've slowly been reprogramming my thoughts and approach to the way I eat. I do see results even when things aren't perfect. Was able to follow the diet in a modified way by combining time groups like purple and blue group at 9 a.m., green and red group at 1 p.m. Noticed that red meat digests much more easily when eaten at lunch rather than dinner. I usually do well the first half of the day, and get a little "hit or miss" in the second half of the day, but it's still working! Finally, a diet that makes sense and doesn't restrict food groups!*

Recipes

Purple Group 7 a.m. – 9 a.m.

Blue Group

Green Group

Red Group

Yellow Group

Orange Group

White Group

Purple Group

BLACKBERRY BREAKFAST SMOOTHIE (7–9 A.M.)

- Soak 1 cup of raw almonds in water overnight (soaking nuts and seeds improves digestibility and reduces anti-nutrients like phytates, lectins, tannins, oxalates)

- 32 oz pressed coconut water, this brand is the best tasting for smoothies, you can substitute a can of light coconut milk if you can't find this

- 1 bag frozen organic blackberries

- Juice of 1 lemon (optional)

- Himalayan salt

- 2 dates or honey (optional)

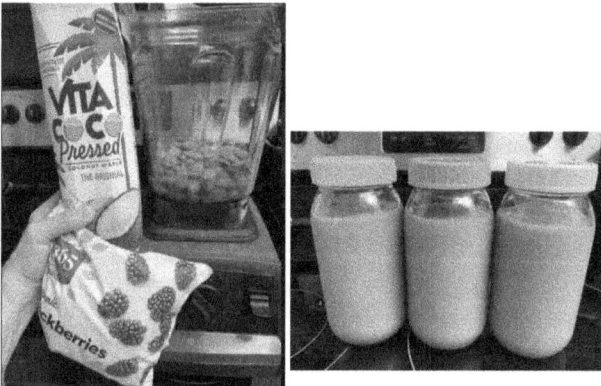

BLUEBERRY LEMON BREAKFAST SMOOTHIE (7-9 A.M.)

- Soak 1 cup of almonds for at least 1 hour

- 1 can of light coconut milk

- 32 oz coconut water

- 1 bag of frozen organic blueberries

- Juice of 1 lemon (this helps preserve it in your fridge for a couple of days, you will get three servings)

- Himalayan salt

- 2 dates or honey (Optional. When I first started the diet I needed the sweetness, but now I add no sweetener because my tastes have changed and yours will too.)

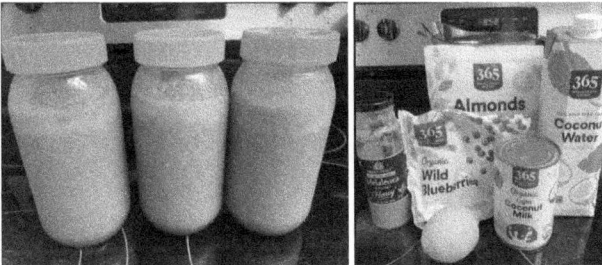

RASPBERRY LIME BREAKFAST SMOOTHIE (7-9 A.M.)

- Soak 1 cup of almonds at least 1 hour

- 1 can light coconut milk and 32 oz coconut water or 32 oz pressed coconut water

- 1 bag frozen organic raspberries

- Juice of 1 lime or lemon (this helps preserve it in your fridge for a couple days, you will get three servings)

- Himalayan salt

- 2 dates or honey (If you need the sweetness, try to do without.)

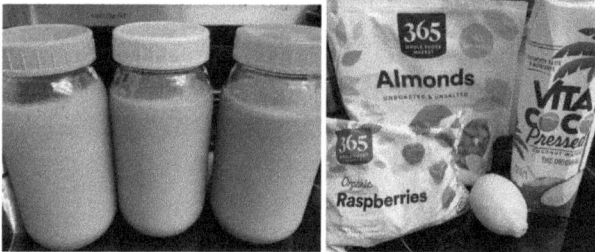

CHERRY-CRANBERRY BREAKFAST SMOOTHIE (7-9 A.M.)

- Soak 1 cup of almonds at least 1 hour

- 32 oz coconut water

- 1 bag frozen organic cranberries

- 1 oz tart cherry juice concentrate

- Himalayan salt

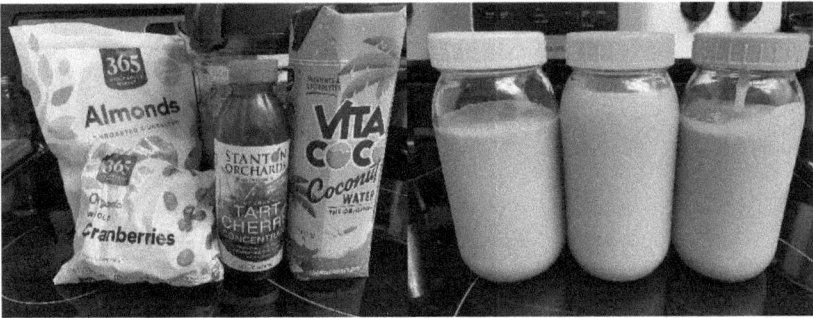

ACAI BERRY SMOOTHIE (7-9 A.M.)

- 1 bag frozen acai, I prefer the unsweetened kind if available, the regular has too much added sugar for my taste

- 1 bag frozen cranberries or other berry

- 1 L coconut water

- Himalayan salt, dates/honey/stevia to taste

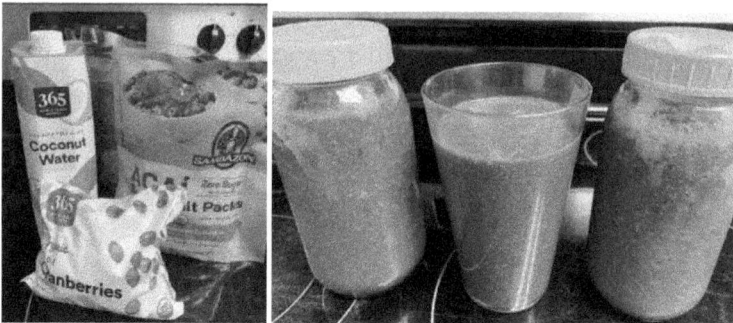

12-OUNCE PURPLE FRUIT SMOOTHIE. FOR A SINGLE SERVING, COMBINE THE FOLLOWING:

- 1 cup blueberries, frozen or fresh

- 1 banana

- 12 almonds

- 2 dates, for sweeter taste

- Coconut water as a base, or plain water or tart cherry juice if you are allergic to nuts

COCOA MOUSSE FOR BREAKFAST (7-9 A.M.) PREPARE THE NIGHT BEFORE AND STORE IN 4 OZ PORTIONS

- This recipe makes 2 portions, you can easily double or triple it

- Add together in blender:

- 1 medium avocado (sometimes you can find avocado chopped and frozen in a bag, this is a huge time saver)

- ¼ cup non-alkalized, non-GMO, cocoa powder

- 2 soaked dates

- Coconut oil, start with 2 tbsp and titrate in up to 2 more tbsp while blending to achieve desired consistency.

- You may add soaked almonds or purple berries (raspberries, cherries) if desired

HOMEMADE CASHEW OR ALMOND BUTTER (7-9 A.M.)

- 2 cups nuts

- 2 tbsp coconut oil

- 1 tsp spices if desired. I like to add chai spice to cashew butter or cinnamon to almonds.

- Combine in blender or food processor at lowest speed and gradually increase until smooth

- For homemade chai spice, combine the following:

- ½ tsp cinnamon

- ½ tsp ground coriander

- ½ tsp ginger

- ½ tsp clove

- ½ tsp cardamon

- Cayenne to taste

Blue Group

CRANBERRY ORANGE RELISH (9–11 A.M.)

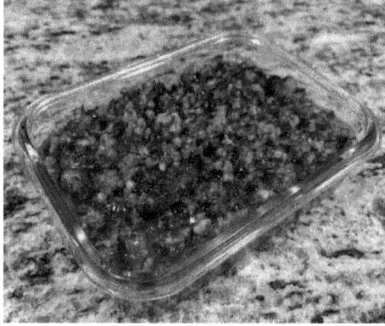

1. In your food processor, combine rind or 1 organic navel orange and its juice with 3-4 tbsp honey / agave / maple syrup until it's almost pureed.

2. Add 1 bag of cleaned organic cranberries and chop at a low setting until you see the desire consistency throughout.

3. Keep in a glass container overnight and enjoy the next morning.

Green Group

GREEN BEAN AMANDINE (11 A.M.– 1 P.M., OR SERVED WITH DINNER)

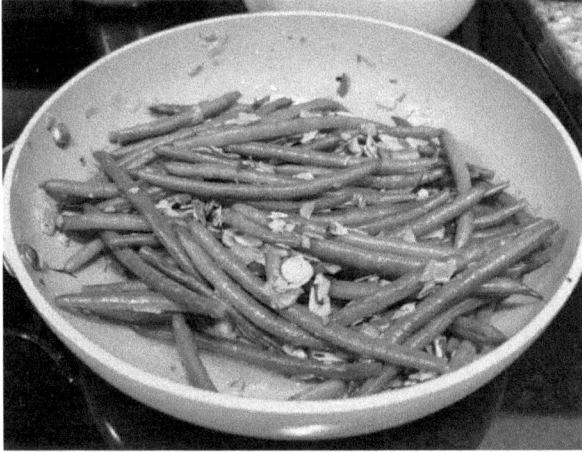

1. In skillet, toast ½ cup sliced almonds in 3 tbsp olive oil, be careful not to burn. Then put in a dish to add back later.

2. In your pan, sauté 2 cloves chopped garlic and 1 large shallot.

3. Add 1 back of green beans and sauté until al dente. Stir in toasted almonds and pull from heat.

MY FAVORITE GREEN SMOOTHIE (11 A.M.– 1 P.M.)

- 1 large coconut water (the coconut water is actually better at this time period than the pressed coconut which is better suited for the 7-9 a.m. electric charge

- ½ bag frozen passion fruit

- Watercress

- Dandelion greens (dandelion leaf is known as a potassium-sparing diuretic, meaning it is high in potassium and works to reduce water retention and bloating. Dandelion greens also provide prebiotic fiber.)

- Swiss chard

- 2 small avocados or 1 medium avocado

- Juice of 1 lime

- Himalayan salt, dash of olive oil

- Honey or dates (optional)

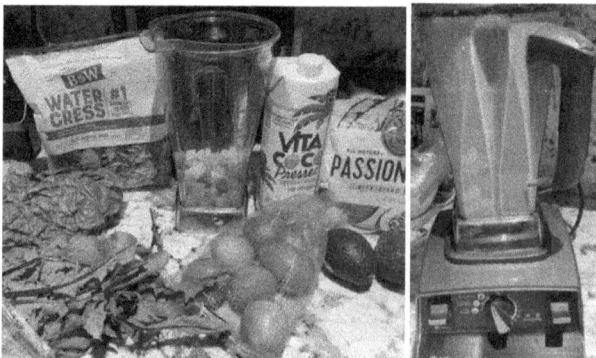

CUCUMBER AVOCADO GREEN SMOOTHIE (11 A.M.– 1 P.M.)

- 1 L coconut water

- Cucumber, I prefer the English kind

- Watercress

- Dandelion greens

- Cilantro

- Parsley

- 2 small avocados

- Juice of 1 lime

- Himalayan salt, dash of olive oil

- If the veggie taste is too *blah* for you, you can use honey or dates to sweeten or another fruit, like kiwi. You can also go the other direction and add jalapeño and extra cilantro.

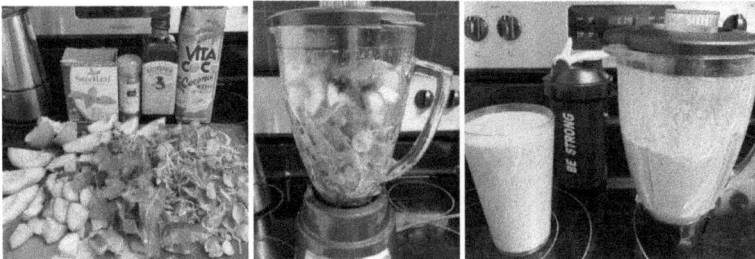

REFRESHING GREEN SMOOTHIE (11 A.M.– 1 P.M.)

- Kale

- Cucumber

- Mint

- Lemon

- Salt

- Dates or honey

- MCT or olive oil (optional)

- 1 L coconut water

- 2 avocados

LEMON APPLE GREEN SMOOTHIE (11 A.M.– 1 P.M.)

- 1 large coconut water

- 2 apples

- 2 avocados

- Kale/spinach/watercress or other leafy green

- Juice of 1 large or 2 small lemons

- Dates/honey/stevia/monk fruit

- Himalayan salt and MCT or olive oil

WATERMELON SALAD (11 A.M. - 1 P.M.)

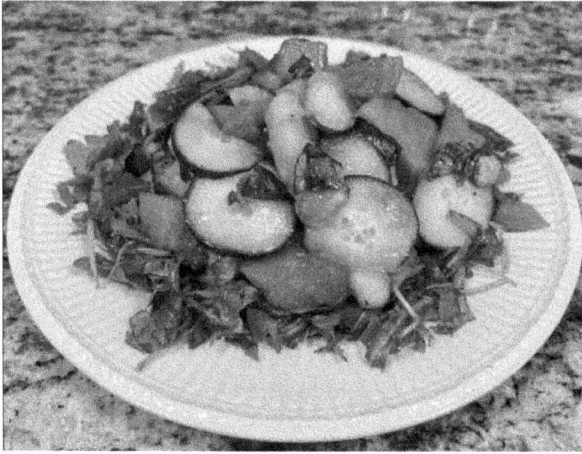

1. **Plate:** Arugula or mixed greens tossed with salt and pepper, olive oil, and balsamic vinegar
2. **Mix in a bowl:**

- Chopped watermelon

- Heirloom tomatoes (try to get the green ones)

- Rainbow radishes

- Cucumber

- Basil, fresh cut

- Salt and pepper to taste

3. **Serve watermelon mixture on top of mixed greens**

SHAVED BALSAMIC CARAMELIZED BRUSSELS SPROUTS (11 A.M. - 1 P.M.)

- Preheat oven to 400°

- Toss together:

- 1 lb. of sliced brussels sprouts

- 2 tbsp olive oil

- 1 tbsp balsamic glaze

- Himalayan salt and fresh ground black pepper

- Place on a cookie sheet lined with parchment paper and bake 25 minutes

- Drizzle with another tbsp balsamic glaze

TABOULEH WITH SPROUTED QUINOA (11 A.M. - 1 P.M.)

- This goes great with kebobs or shawarma for a late lunch ~ 2 p.m.~

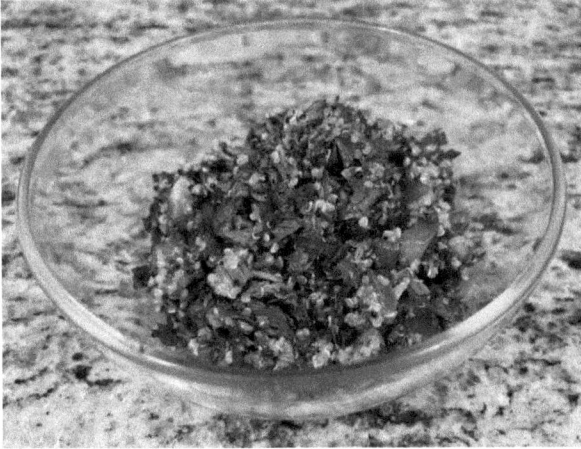

- Dice ¾ lb ripe plum tomatoes, season with 1 tsp salt and transfer to a colander to allow the juices to drain; you will use the juice later to make the quinoa. This is an important step as it keeps your tabbouleh from being soggy.

- Chop 2 cups / 2 bunches of Italian flat leaf parsley and season with 1 tsp salt. Transfer to a bowl lined with paper towel to absorb excess moisture.

- Cook ½ cup dry sprouted quinoa with the tomato water and allow it to cool in the refrigerator. Sprouted grains can be eaten in the red group as well as the white group because the sprouting process gives the grain a thermic energetic quality in addition to the insular energetic quality.

In a large mixing bowl, combine:

- Tomatoes

- Parsley

- 1 cup chopped mint leaves

- 1-2 scallions finely chopped

- ¼ cup + olive oil

- 2 tbsp fresh lemon juice

- ¼ tsp coriander

- ¼ tsp cinnamon

- Salt and black pepper to taste

BORSCHT (1-3 P.M.)

This took about an hour of prep time due to chopping all the vegetables, it has a very distinct flavor and a high nutritional value. We have a large Russian population in Miami. I tried to include diverse food choices in the 7-Day Reset but you can swap out items according to taste.

- Sauté in large pot:

- 2 Tbsp olive oil

- 1 lb bison or beef stew meat

- 1 large onion

- 4 garlic cloves

- Add in, bring to a boil, and then simmer 30 minutes:

- 1 qt beef bone broth

- 4 carrots

- 4 celery stalks

- 2 medium beets, shredded

- 1 cup cabbage, add in the last 10 minutes

- 1 russet potato

- ½ tsp salt

- ½ tsp pepper

- ½ tsp allspice (I had to substitute cinnamon, nutmeg, and clove)

- ½ tsp cumin

- ½ tsp paprika

- Dash cayenne

- 2 bay leaves

- 3 tbsp tomato paste or 1 fresh tomato diced

- Turn off heat and stir in:

- 6 tbsp apple cider vinegar or lemon juice

- Garnish with fresh chopped dill

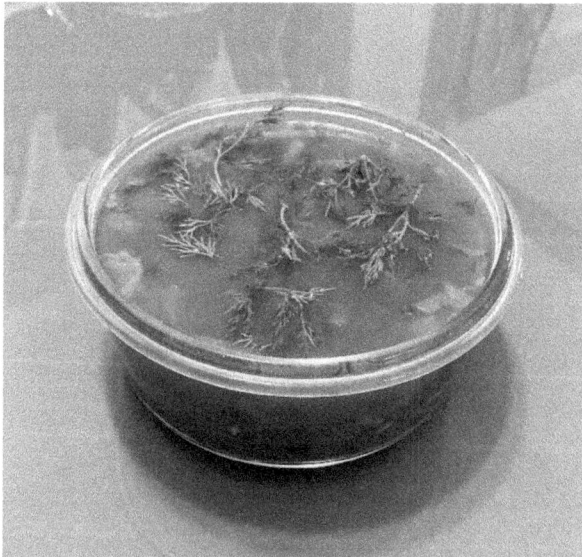

CORN (ANY VEGETABLE) SOUP (3-5 P.M. OR 11 A.M. - 1 P.M. IF MADE WITH GREEN VEGGIES)

- Puree in food processor or blender and simmer 20 minutes

- 1 lb frozen roasted corn, thawed (substitute potatoes and leeks or broccoli, butternut squash, etc.)

- 1 qt bone broth

- ½ tsp thyme or substitute herb such as tarragon

- ¼ tsp white or black pepper

- ¼ cup chopped onion or shallots

- Salt if needed

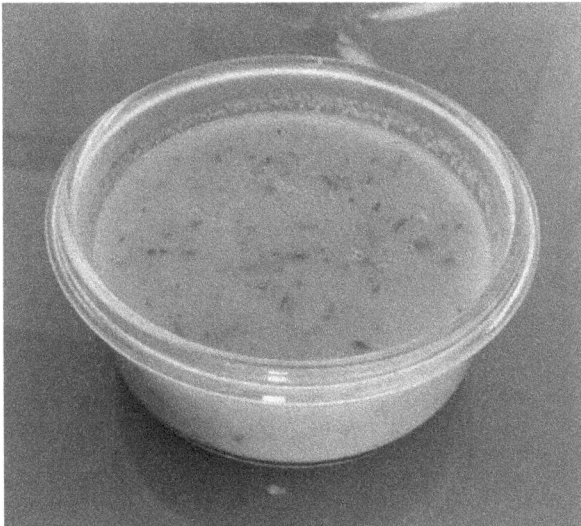

VEGAN PESTO

- 1 bunch basil, about a cup and a half chopped

- ½ cup raw cashews or walnuts

- 1 4 or 6 oz bag pine nuts

- 1 cup olive oil

- Himalayan salt and fresh ground pepper

- Pulse ingredients in food processor

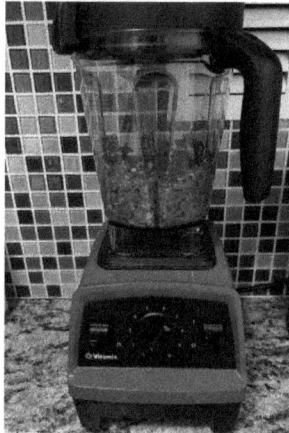

Red Group

GREEK LAMB SHANK (3-5 P.M. OR 6-7 P.M.)

- This has a 25 min prep time + 2.5-3 hours in oven, depending on the size of your shanks

- 1. Mix in a glass baking dish and cover with foil, set aside:

- 1 lb organic baby red potatoes cut into quarters

- ½ jar kalamata olives sliced lengthwise

- 1 fresh lemon juiced and then diced

- 2 tsp oregano

- Salt and pepper to taste

- Olive oil

- Enough chicken bone broth to make ¼ inch deep in the pan

- 2. In a large Ziploc bag, combine 1 tsp of each of the following:

- 1 tap salt

- 1 tsp garlic powder

- 1 tsp basil

- 2 tsp oregano

- ½ tsp cinnamon

- 1 tsp black pepper

- 1 tsp parsley

- 1 tsp rosemary

- 1 tsp dill

- 1 tsp marjoram

- 1 tsp thyme

- ½ tsp nutmeg

- 3. Shake and add your lamb shanks

- 4. Put lamb shanks in glass baking dish along with the other ½ jar of kalamata olives, and another diced lemon. Cover with foil and put in oven at 300°.

- 5. Go to the gym, pick up the kids, have a meeting...come back in like 2-2.5 hours (depending on the size of your lamb shanks).

- 6. Throw the potatoes in the oven and crank it up to 400° F for 30 minutes.

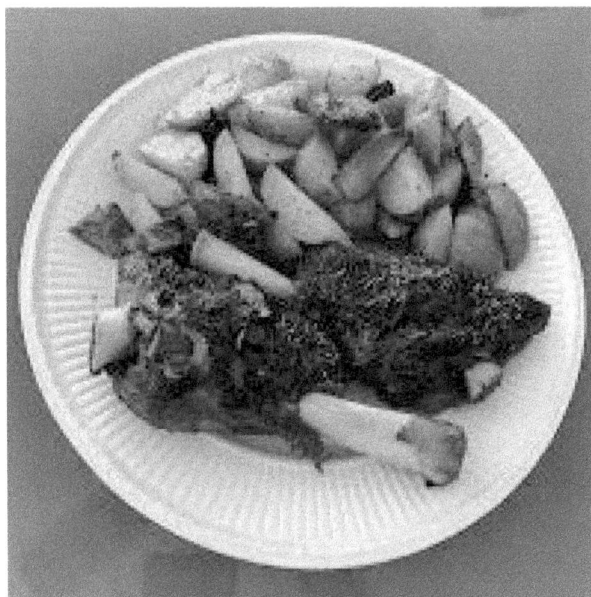

CHIMICHURRI SAUCE

- 1 cup parsley

- 1 cup cilantro

- ½ cup olive oil

- 2 garlic cloves

- ¼ cup apple cider vinegar or lemon juice

- ½-1 tsp Himalayan salt

- ½ tsp black pepper

- Crushed red pepper flakes to taste

- Pulse ingredients in a food processor, blender or Vitamix, top your grilled steaks or seafood with it

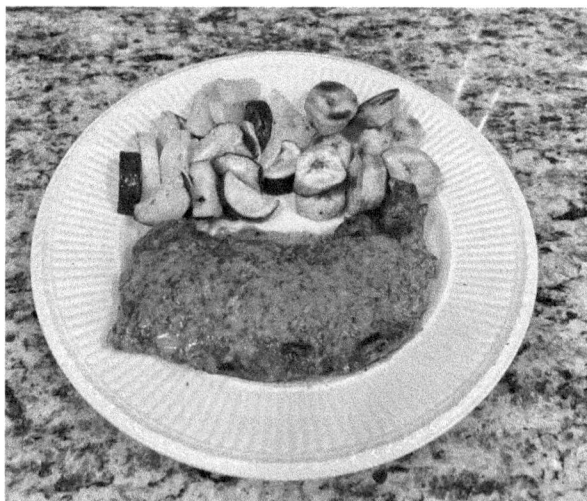

BAKED HALIBUT, WHITE ASPARAGUS, AND SWISS CHARD WITH HOLLANDAISE (1-5 P.M. OR 6-7 P.M.)

This has a 30-minute prep time if you are actively trying to lose weight, and a 45-minute prep time if you make the hollandaise sauce.

1. On a cookie sheet, lay down parchment paper, halibut, asparagus (please trim the bottoms and side leaflets to make sure you don't eat sand later), and Swiss chard.

2. Drizzle olive oil, salt, and pepper over everything; squeeze a little lemon juice and fresh herbs on top of fish.

3. Bake at 400° F for 20-25 minutes, depending on the thickness of your filet.

4. Pull out of oven and let it rest.

5. Over a double boiler, melt ½ stick of butter.

6. Add in 2 tbsp Dijon mustard and juice of 1 large lemon.

7. Whisk in egg yolks slowly.

8. Plate your fish and cover with hollandaise, dust with paprika.

9. Enjoy! This meal is a party in your mouth!

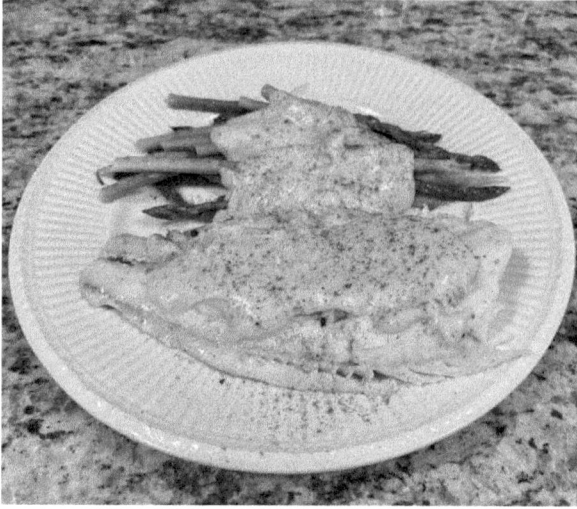

ROSEMARY LAMB SHOULDER OR RACK OF LAMB WITH ROOT VEGETABLES (1-5 P.M.)

This is good for an early dinner closer to 5 p.m. which is ideal if you plan to have dessert around 7 p.m. Even if your goal is to lose weight, you are permitted to have cake on holidays!

1. Preheat oven to 400°

2. Line one cookie sheet with parchment paper and lay down lamb; dust with salt and pepper to taste and rosemary (I prefer fresh, but dried will do the trick)

3. Line a second cookie sheet with parchment paper for the root vegetables. I like to get a bag of frozen veggies to save time. Drizzle with olive oil and season with salt, black pepper, and rosemary

4. Bake for about 25-30 minutes, be careful not to overcook the lamb

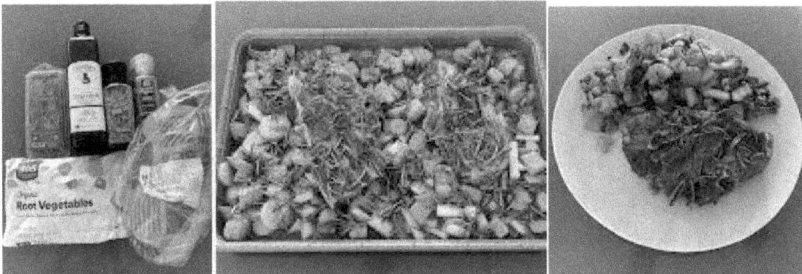

CHICKEN BREAST WITH KIMCHEE AND TAMARI AND BOK CHOY WITH COCONUT AMINOS (1-3 P.M. OR 6-7 P.M. IF YOU WANT TO ADD COCONUT BASMATI AS A SIDE)

- Preheat oven to 400°

- Break up baby bok choy leaves and toss with 1 tbsp coconut oil and 2 tbsp coconut aminos, place on parchment paper lined cookie sheet and bake approximately 30 minutes, stirring once after 20 minutes

- Trim and dice chicken breasts

- Sauté chicken in coconut oil and tamari, make sure the oil is hot, so you get a good sear

- When fully cooked, pull off heat and add kimchee–add siracha if you like more heat

- Allow chicken to rest while bok choy is getting crispy greens in the oven

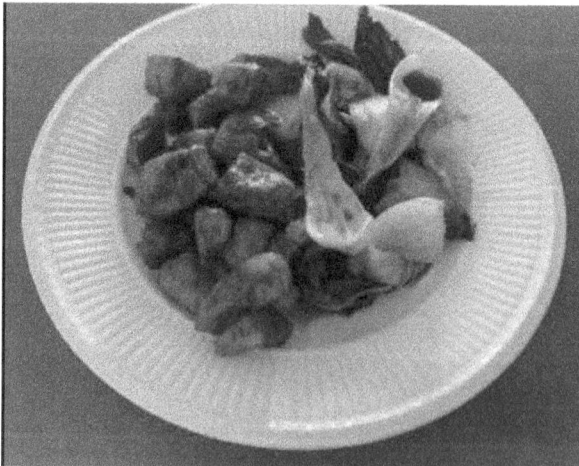

BEEF/BUFFALO STEW (1-3 P.M. ANY DAY OR 6-7 P.M. ON FRIDAYS)

- Sauté 1 cup chopped onion and 1 lb beef/buffalo chuck

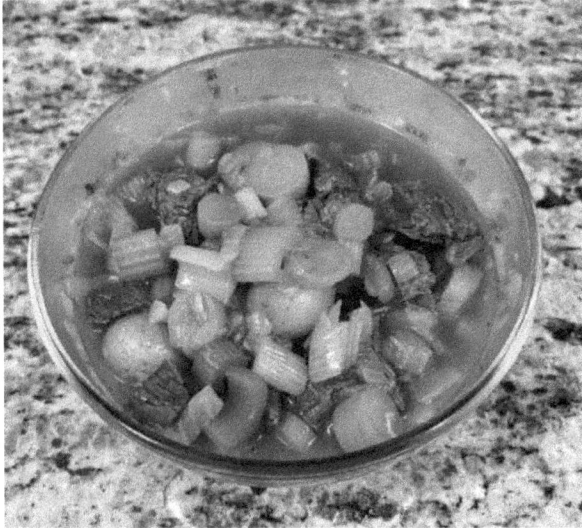

- Add to meat mixture in pot and cook together 30 minutes:

- 1 cup celery

- 1 cup carrots

- 2-3 cups fingerling potatoes

- 1 cup red or white wine

- 1 qt beef bone broth

- 1 bay leaf

CHICKEN TOMATILLO SOUP (1-5 P.M.)

- Sauté 1 lb chicken breasts chopped into bite size pieces in olive oil, with 3-4 garlic cloves and 1 chopped onion

- Combine in pot and cook approximately 30 minutes:

- 4 cups chicken bone broth

- 4 cups chopped tomatillo

- Salt and pepper to taste

- Pull off heat and stir in:

- 1 cup chopped cilantro

- Juice of 2 limes

- Top with chopped avocado and cilantro, serve with plantain chips if desired

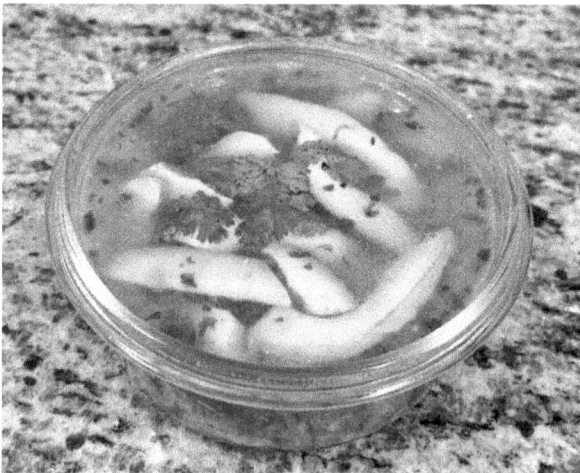

LEMON POACHED COD (1-3 P.M. IF EATEN ALONE OR 6-7 P.M. IF EATEN WITH PASTA/POTATOES/RICE)

- Sear on both sides in olive oil, 4 x 4–6-ounce pieces of cod

- Add in:

- ½ cup chicken bone broth

- ½ cup white wine or vermouth

- Salt and pepper to taste

- Cover with lid and cook 7-8 minutes max

BEEF STEAK AU POIVRE WITH SAUTEED FENNEL AND LEEKS (1-3 P.M. OR 6-7 P.M. ON FRIDAYS)

- Combine in frying pan:

- 1.5 lbs. grass fed beef or buffalo, diced, and seared in 2 tbsp olive oil

- Add in and sauté together:

- 1 clove garlic

- ¼ cup shallots

- 1 tbsp black peppercorns

- Stir in and simmer 1 hour:

- ½ cup red wine

- 2 cups beef bone broth with 1 tbsp of cornstarch

- Clean and slice 1 leek and 1 fennel bulb, and sauté in a pan with 2 tbsp olive oil, salt, and pepper to taste

- Prepare mashed potatoes. I prefer organic russet potatoes because they have as much potassium as a banana. I leave the skins on and mix them with salted grass-fed butter.

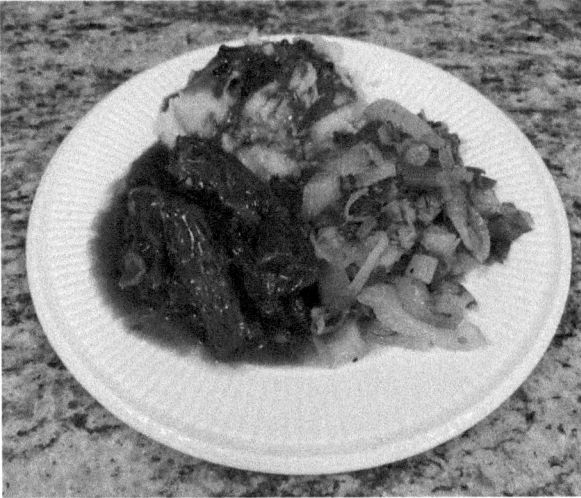

Yellow Group

BAKED CAULIFLOWER (3-5 P.M. OR 6-7 P.M.)

- 1 head of cauliflower cut into florets

- 2 tbsp olive oil

- 2 garlic cloves

- Salt and pepper to taste

- *If you would like a more spicey version, add 1 tsp smoked paprika and 1 tsp turmeric

- Chopped fresh parsley for garnish

- Roast 20 minutes at 425°, toss/flip cauliflower and roast an additional 5 minutes. Toss with wing sauce for vegetarian "chicken wings."

COLOMBIAN CHICKEN SANCOCHO SOUP (3-5 P.M. OR 6-7 P.M.)

This makes a great dinner on a cold rainy day, especially if feeling under the weather. This took about an hour of prep time due to chopping all the vegetables, it has a very distinct flavor and a high nutritional value. We have a small Colombian population in Miami. I tried to include diverse food choices in the 7-Day Reset but you can swap out items according to taste.

- Sauté 2 tbsp olive oil, 1 medium onion, and 3 cloves of chopped garlic in a pot

- Add 6+ diced chicken thighs and sauté until cooked thoroughly

- Add 2 medium or 1 large, chopped tomato

- 3-4 chopped Yukon Gold potatoes

- Yucca, diced

- 1 green plantain, diced

- 2 quarts chicken bone broth

- ½ tsp cumin

- Salt and pepper to taste

- Boil 40 min, add 6 corn cobs cut in half and boil additional 15 minutes

- Pull off heat and add ½ cup chopped cilantro and juice of 2-3 limes

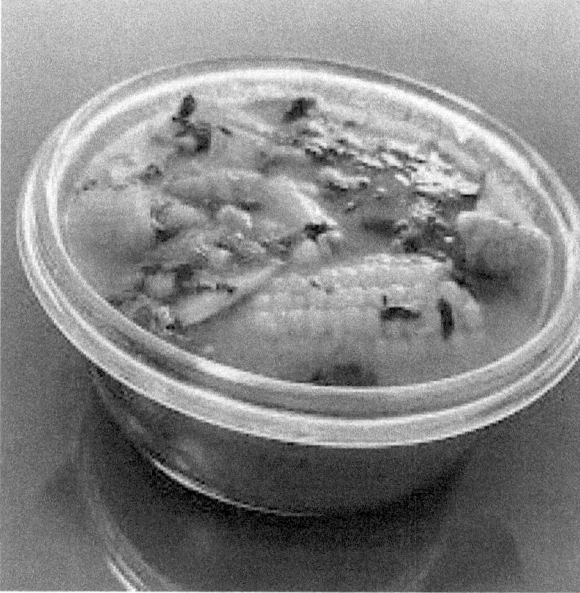

BASIL QUINOA SALAD (3-5 P.M.)

- This is best digested between 3-5 p.m. (or on Wednesdays outside of that timeframe because of the raw non-green veggies)

- Prepare 1 cup dry sprouted quinoa as directed on the package, you may substitute some of the water for white wine or bone broth if desired. Remember that sprouted grains also gain a thermic energy so you can utilize the nutrients during the red time 1-3 p.m.

- Slice 1 small bag of sweet peppers and sauté in olive oil.

- Chop and combine in a large bowl:

- 1 ½ cups kale or arugula

- 1 ½ cups basil leaf

- 1-pint yellow grape or heirloom tomatoes cut into halves

- ½ jar kalamata olives chopped small

- 1 can of hearts of palm sliced thin

- Juice of 1 lemon or 2 tbsp balsamic glaze

- Salt and pepper to taste

- Quinoa (chilled)

- Sweet peppers in olive oil mix

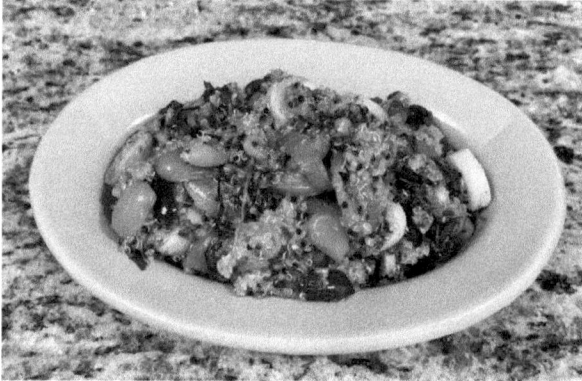

PACIFIC HALIBUT WITH BUTTERNUT SQUASH PUREE AND PEAS AND CARROTS (3-5 P.M. OR 6-7 P.M.)

- Preheat oven to 400°

- Cook 2 diced shallots in chicken bone broth until clear, add diced butternut squash, 1 tsp tarragon, ½ tsp sage, ½ tsp white pepper and garlic salt to taste

- Place fish on cookie sheet lined with parchment paper and season with olive oil, juice of 1 lemon, salt, and pepper. Bake approximately 15 minutes or until flaky.

- When squash is fully cooked, puree in food processor.

- Do not overcook peas and carrots, I like mine with grass-fed butter, salt, and pepper

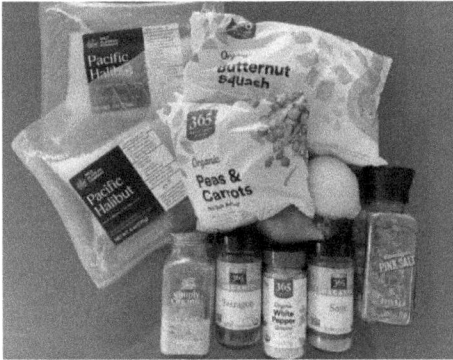

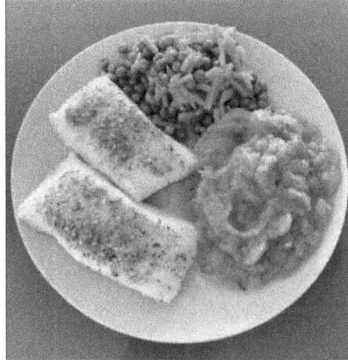

MOQUECA (BRAZILIAN FISH STEW) (2-5 P.M. PLAIN OR 6-7 P.M. IF SERVED WITH RICE)

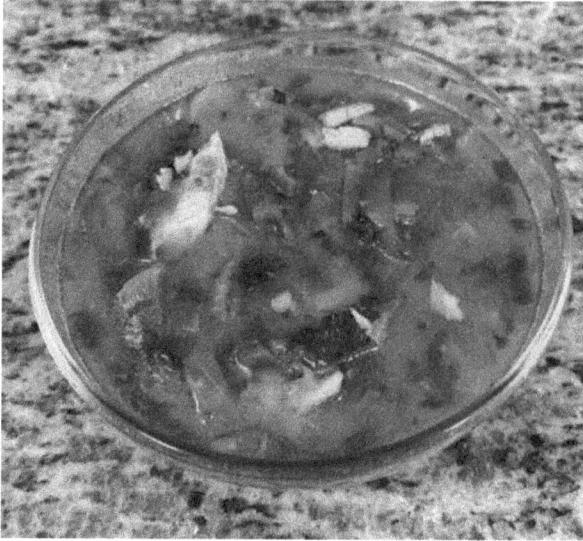

- Season 2 pounds of whitefish like mahi-mahi or cod in the juice of 1 lime, salt, and pepper, and put in the fridge for 15 min while you chop veggies

- Sautee 3 cloves of garlic in olive oil a couple of minutes

- Add 1 can of diced tomatoes on top (I prefer the fire roasted) and then layer 1 sliced onion and 3 bell peppers sliced (1 yellow, 1 red, 1 green), and 1 serrano or jalapeño (optional)

- Layer fish on top, then add 1 small bunch each of chopped parsley and cilantro, and then sprinkle 1 tsp of ground coriander, salt, and pepper to taste

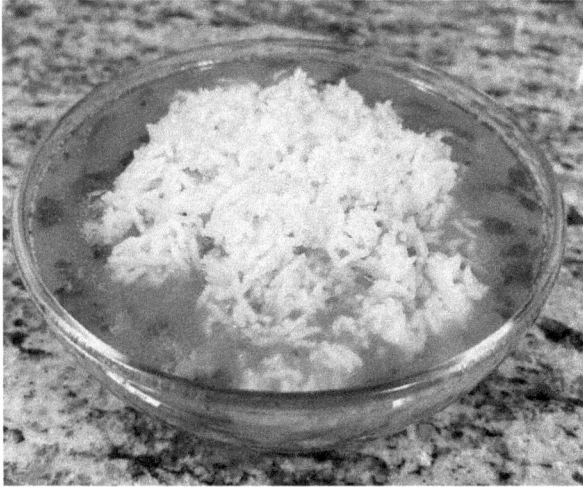

- Cover with a lid and simmer on medium heat for 15-20 minutes until fish is cooked, onions are clear, peppers are soft, etc. Avoid the temptation to stir the pot like a maniac, you will just break up the fish.

- Add 1 can of coconut milk (look for one that doesn't have guar gum) and 2 tbsp tomato paste

- Serve with salad if you are eating this earlier in the day or with rice if you are eating this for dinner. Because of the peppers, it is best digested on a Wednesday if you are having it 6-7 p.m.

Orange Group

LENTIL SOUP WITH GINGER AND TURMERIC (5-6 P.M.)

- Soak 1 cup lentils overnight and add 1/4 tsp baking soda to water.

- Rinse in fresh water and combine in a large pot:

- Chopped celery and carrots, approximately 1 cup total

- 4 cloves garlic

- 3 cups bone broth or water

- Add small amount of grated ginger and/or turmeric, then cook until soft.

I like to cook in bone broth to add collagen and more nutrients.

- You can also add ½ tsp each of cumin, cinnamon, and coriander

- Add Celtic salt or sea salt to taste

- Garnish with lemon

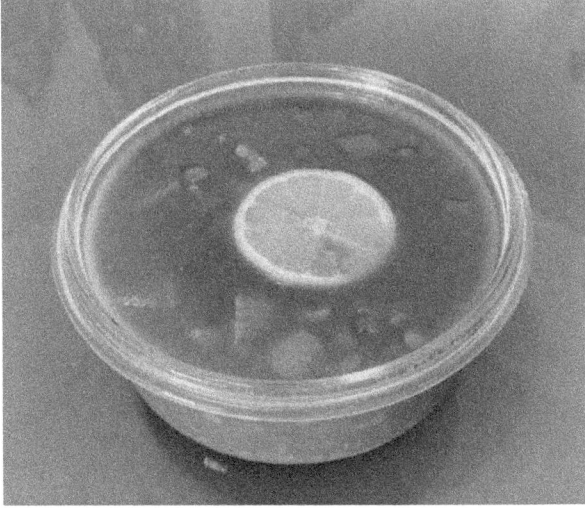

HUMMUS (5-6 P.M.)

- 1 cup cooked garbanzo beans

- 6 tbs olive or coconut oil

- 1 garlic clove

- Salt to taste

- 3 tbs tahini

- 1 small lemon

Pre-soak beans overnight in 1 tsp of baking soda or another degassing herb. Cook beans well and strain juice but save to add in later while mixing to reduce the consistency. Put half the amount of garbanzo beans in the blender with the oil and slowly mix in juice from cooking. If it is too runny, add a little more bean, add the tahini, slowly add lemon to taste, and finish with salt. I eat this with crudité: romaine lettuce, yellow pepper strips, carrots, and celery; do this instead of white foods like pita bread, if you want to reduce body fat.

YELLOW LENTIL DAHL (5-6 P.M.)

- Sauté in a large pot:

- 2 tbsp olive or coconut oil

- 1 onion diced

- 2 cloves garlic

- Add to mixture and simmer 25 min until liquid is absorbed:

- 2 cups bone broth

- 1 ½ cups yellow lentils, rinsed

- 1 tsp Himalayan salt

- 1 tsp turmeric

- 1 tsp ground cumin (if you have cumin seeds, sauté 3 tbsp with the onions and garlic instead)

- Red pepper flakes to taste

- Garnish with fresh chopped cilantro

White Group

**SOFRITO MARINATED BUFFALO RIBEYE WITH
COCONUT RICE (FRIDAY 6-7 P.M.)
30-MINUTE COOK TIME**

- The night before, marinate your ribeye or tenderloins in Worcestershire and sofrito sauce, I like the brand called "Sky Valley."

- Get a medium pot and combine basmati rice, 1 can light coconut milk and chicken bone broth, bring to a boil and then reduce to simmer.

- Either on a grill or heat a pan with olive oil to sear the steaks, cook to desire temperature.

- Buffalo filet steaks are so delicious and tender. You may be able to save money by ordering from *Butcher Box* or another delivery service; they deliver to your doorstep.

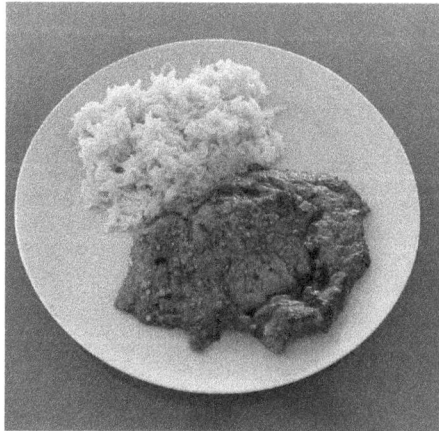

BOWTIE PASTA WITH LOBSTER "CREAM" SAUCE (6-7 P.M.)

- 1 lb diced lobster, sometimes this comes pre-seasoned from the grocer's seafood department

- ¼ tsp nutmeg

- Seafood seasoning to taste (I like low-country boil seasoning mix, use what you have)

- ¼ - ½ cup fresh dill, tarragon, and Italian flat leaf parsley chopped

- 2 tbsp butter

- 1 can light coconut milk

- Salt and pepper to taste

- In a medium-sized pot, melt 2 tbsp butter, add nutmeg, salt, pepper, seafood seasoning.

- Whisk in coconut milk and allow to heat thoroughly but do not boil.

- Stir in lobster and fresh green spices, do not overcook lobster.

- Serve with gluten-free bowtie pasta and enjoy pasta with "cream" sauce that doesn't leave you feeling bloated.

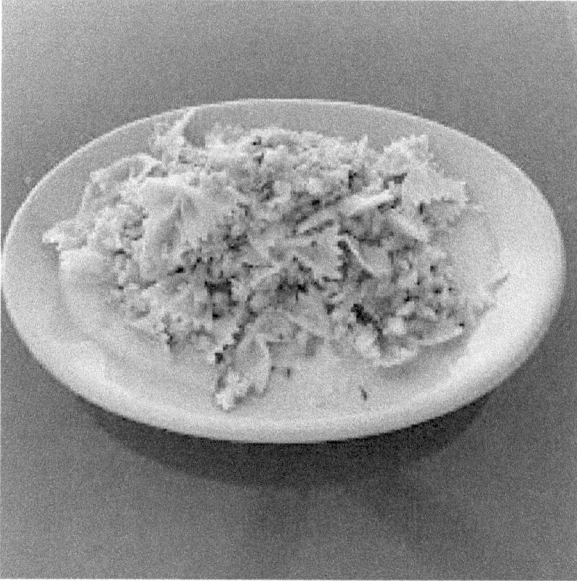

SHRIMP ORZO (6-7 P.M.)

- Combine in large pot and cook until orzo is al dente:

- 1 cup gluten-free orzo

- 1 qt chicken bone broth

- ½ cup white wine, I like sauvignon blanc

- 2 cloves garlic chopped

- Salt and pepper to taste

- Add in:

- 1 lb shrimp

- ½ cup chopped parsley

SHRIMP SCAMPI PASTA (6-7 P.M.)

- Boil your water for pasta. My favorite brand is *Jovial*

- In a pan sauté:

- 1 lb of shrimp, I like bigger shrimp for this meal

- 2 tbsp olive oil

- 2-3 cloves garlic

- ½ cup chopped fresh parsley

- Salt and pepper to taste, sometimes I like to combine white and black pepper in this dish

- When the shrimp are fully cooked, pull off the heat and add the juice of 1 lemon and 2-3 tbsp grass-fed butter

- Toss together and enjoy

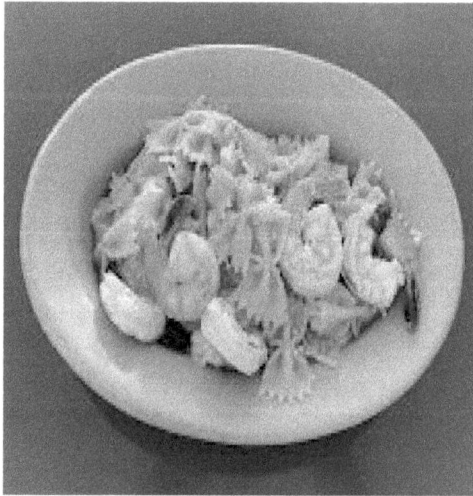

ARTICHOKE CHICKEN PASTA (6-7 P.M.)

- Sauté together in a medium frying pan:

- 2 tbsp olive oil

- 4 chicken breasts or 6 thighs diced

- 2 tbsp rosemary

- 1 tbsp sage

- 1 tsp white pepper

- 1 small clove of garlic finely minced

- 4 oz chopped prosciutto or bacon

- In a 2nd frying pan, spread out 2+ tbsp olive oil and take a can of quartered artichokes and place them in the pan choke side down, add salt and pepper to taste; brown on 1 side and then turn over

- Start to boil a large pot of water for pasta

- In the pan with the artichokes, add ½ jar of kalamata olives sliced in quarters lengthwise and ½ jar capers

- Once the chicken is more than halfway cooked, add a small bag of pine nuts

- When chicken is fully cooked and pine nuts are toasted, pull off heat and add to the artichoke mix

- Then toss with gluten-free penne or fusilli pasta–voila!

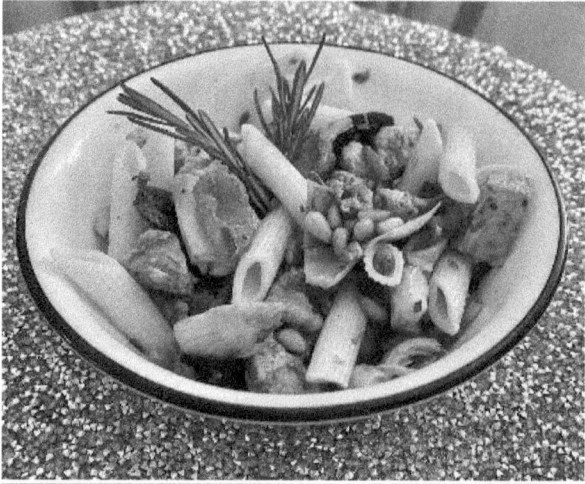

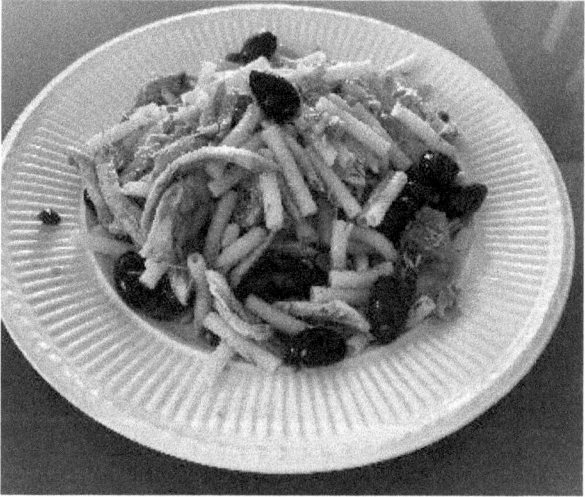

JAMAICAN JERK SOCKEYE SALMON WITH MILLET AND PEAS (6-7 P.M.)

- Preheat oven to 375°

- In a medium-sized pot, sauté millet in olive oil until toasted–be careful not to burn

- Add chicken bone broth, a little bit of jerk seasoning, bring to a boil and then simmer for 30 minutes

- Place the salmon skin side down on a cookie sheet lined with parchment paper, dust with Jamaican Jerk seasoning, and bake 20 minutes

- In a small pot, slightly boil your peas and carrots, do not overcook (I like mine with butter, but I am trying to maintain my weight, not lose weight.)

- Millet is a great gluten-free alternative to couscous; it's high in calcium and insoluble fiber (prebiotics)

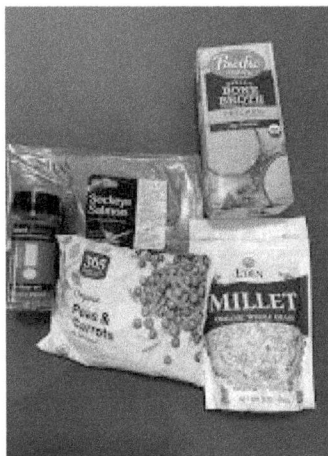

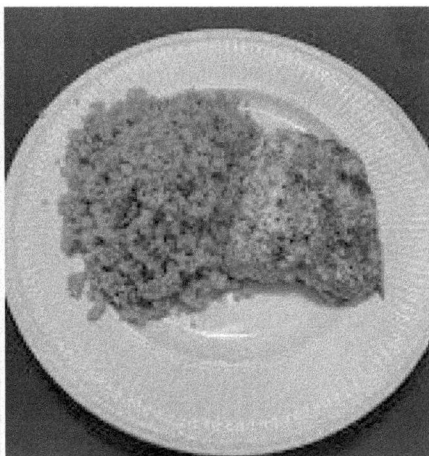

VEGGIE STIR FRY (FEEDS TWO PEOPLE, DOUBLE THE RECIPE FOR YOUR FAMILY) 6-7 P.M.

- Pick three vegetables: snow pea pods, carrots, mushrooms, broccoli, bok choy, bamboo shoots, water chestnuts

- Pick a protein like ½ pound of shrimp or 2 chicken breasts, or 4 chicken thighs

- Sauté together until the garlic is cooked, stir often, don't burn

- 2 garlic cloves

- 1 tbsp ginger fresh or 1 tsp ginger powder

- 1 tbsp coconut oil

- Add the veggies and cook until they are al dente (no soggy veggies please) and set aside

- Add in your protein and sauté until they're cooked thoroughly

- Mix together ¼ cup water, ¼ cup tamari or soy sauce, and 1 tbsp cornstarch, then add to the proteins cooking in the pan, this should make a sauce

- Add the veggies back in and remove the pan from heat

- Serve with 1 cup of rice maximum, <1 cup if trying to lose weight. I like the sauce from the stir fry on my rice but that may not be enough flavor for your taste buds. You may season additionally with *Bragg* or coconut aminos, gluten-free tamari, or nutritional yeast.

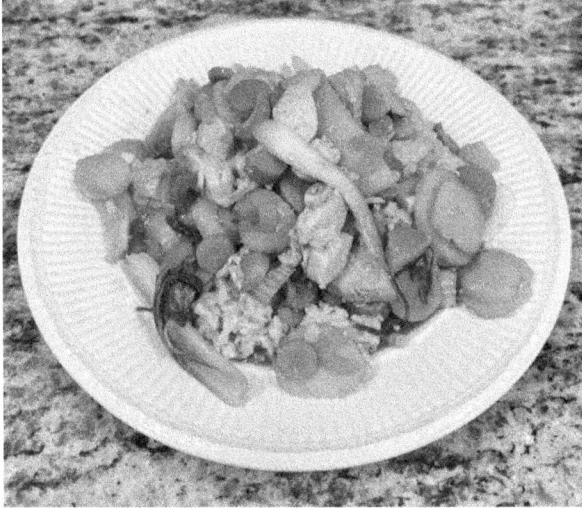

CHICKEN FAJITAS (FEEDS TWO PEOPLE, DOUBLE THE RECIPE FOR YOUR FAMILY) 6-7 P.M.

- Cut 1 pound of chicken breast into bite-size pieces

- In a skillet, heat 1 tbsp coconut or avocado oil with

- 1 tsp cumin

- 1 tsp paprika

- ½ tsp garlic powder or 2 cloves garlic

- ½ tsp oregano

- ½ tsp black pepper

- ¼ tsp cayenne (optional, may need more or less depending on your preference)

- ½ tsp Himalayan salt

- Add diced chicken and sauté until meat is firm

- Add 1 sliced bell pepper and 1 sliced onion

- Mix together ¼ cup of water, juice of 1 lime, and 1 tbsp cornstarch and stir into sauce to thicken, then remove from heat

- Serve with gluten-free tortillas, pico de gallo, and guacamole

- Optional: plantain chips to dip the extra guac and pico

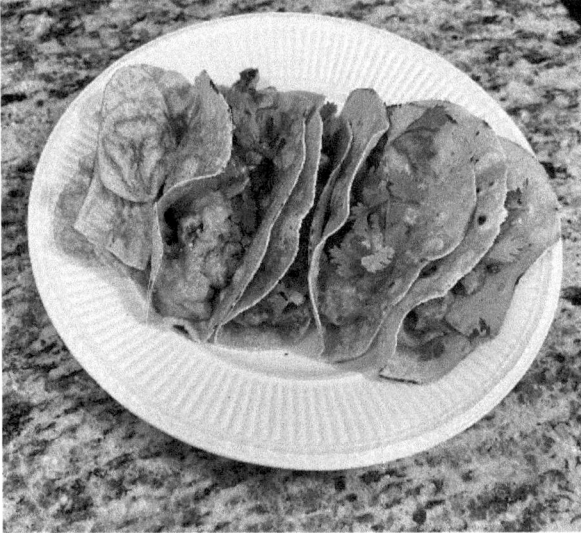

GINGER WASABI HALIBUT WITH COCONUT BASMATI RICE (6-7 P.M.)

- Preheat oven to 400°

- Prepare rice as directed on the stove, substituting some of the water for bone broth and coconut cream

- Put halibut on cookie sheet lines with parchment paper and cover with wasabi paste and minced ginger

- Bake 15 minutes or until flaky, I seasoned with Himalayan salt, but you can use tamari or aminos

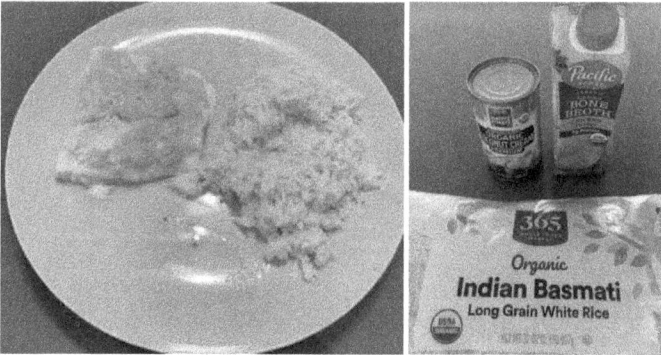

SWEET AND SOUR CHICKEN (OR SHRIMP) WITH COCONUT BASMATI RICE (6-7 P.M.)

- Prepare basmati rice as directed on the package, substitute 1 can of light coconut milk and chicken bone broth for water. Roughly 1 cup of dry rice to 1 ½ -2 cups of liquid.

- Dice 1 pound of chicken breast or thighs and marinate in 1 tbsp gluten-free tamari or soy sauce.

- Prepare Sweet and Sour Sauce: Combine in a saucepan and bring to a boil:

- 1 can of crushed pineapple with juice, 2 tbsp siracha or more depending on your preference, 2 tbsp tamari/soy/ fish sauce, 2 tbsp vinegar, and 2 tbsp lime juice

- Stir in 1 tbsp cornstarch with ¼ cup water (premixed) to thicken the sauce and remove from heat

- Chop 2 garlic cloves, 1 carrot, 1 celery stalk, and ½ onion, and sauté in a large pan with 1 tbsp coconut oil

- Add 1 can of bamboo shoots and diced chicken, and cook thoroughly

- Add Sweet and Sour pineapple sauce to chicken and vegetable mixture and serve over rice

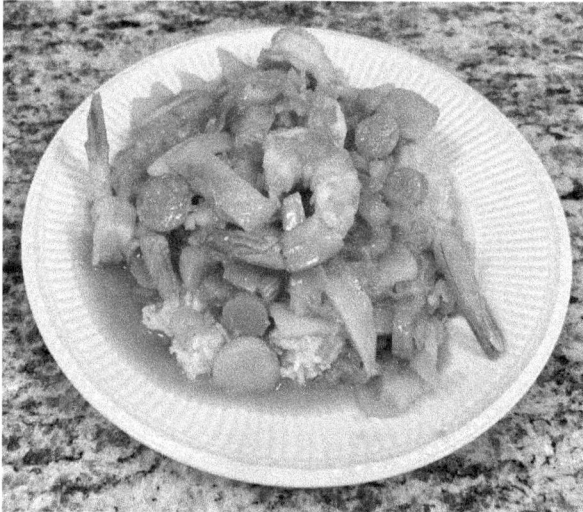

DIJON DILL COHO SALMON WITH OVEN-ROASTED DILL POTATOES (3-5 P.M. OR 6-7 P.M.)

- Preheat oven to 400°

- Toss potatoes with olive oil, fresh dill, Himalayan salt, and fresh ground black pepper

- Place on cookie sheet lined with parchment paper and bake approximately 30 minutes, it depends on the size of your potatoes, I like making them bite-size, so they cook faster.

- Place Coho skin side down on cookie sheet lined with parchment paper, coat with Dijon mustard, fresh dill, and capers. Throw into the oven approximately 15 minutes, depending on how well you like them done. Frozen fish does not have parasites so you can leave it more medium if you prefer.

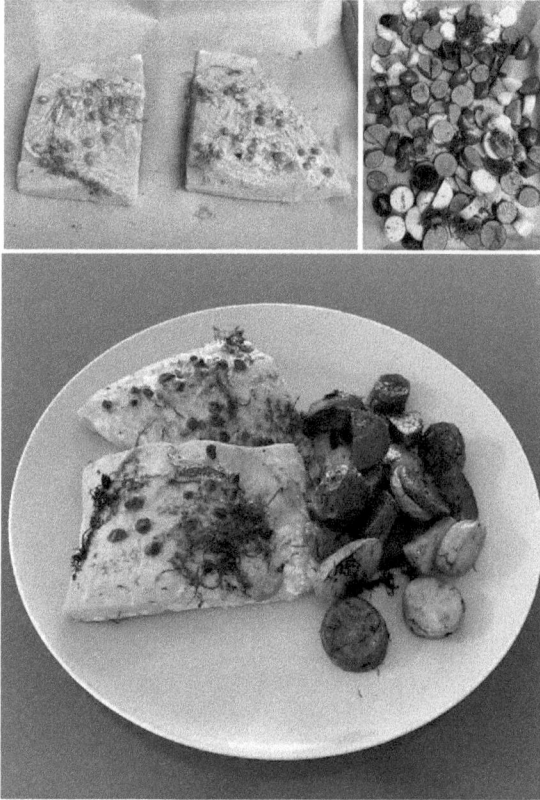

ROCKFISH WITH VEGAN PESTO GNOCCHI (6-7 P.M.)

- Preheat oven to 400°

- Place fish on cookie sheet lines with parchment paper and season with thyme (fresh is best), paprika, Himalayan salt and fresh ground pepper. Drizzle with olive oil and juice of 1 lemon

- Bake 15 minutes or until done, depends on how thick your filets are

- Prepare gnocchi as directed and toss with vegan pesto, this brand of frozen pasta is high in protein which I love

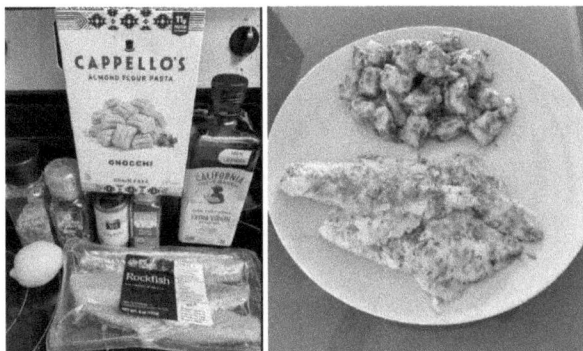

LOBSTER RISOTTO (6-7 P.M.)

- Combine in a pot and boil 25 minutes:

- 2 tbsp fresh tarragon

- Salt, fresh ground black pepper and white pepper to taste

- 1 cup white wine or ½ cup dry vermouth

- 1 small onion or 2-3 medium shallots

- 1 quart chicken bone broth

- 2 cups arborio rice

- 1 stick grass-fed butter (you can make it with ½ stick of butter if you are trying to lose weight)

- Turn off burner and add in 1 lb cooked lobster meat (you can substitute crab or crawfish)

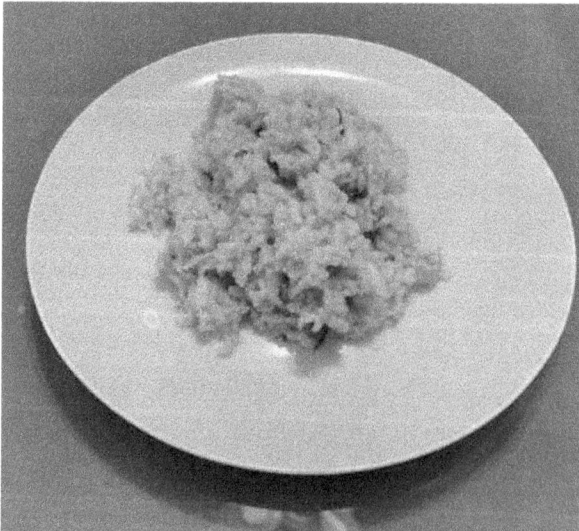

CHICKEN OR VEAL FRICASSEE (3-5 P.M. OR 6-7 P.M.)

- Sear on both sides in butter or olive oil, 2 lbs. Chicken thighs or veal

- Add in and sauté:

- 1 onion and 1 fennel bulb

- Add in and simmer 25 minutes:

- 2 cups chicken bone broth

- 2 cups vegetables: fingerling potatoes, carrots, parsnips, etc.

- Garnish with fresh parsley

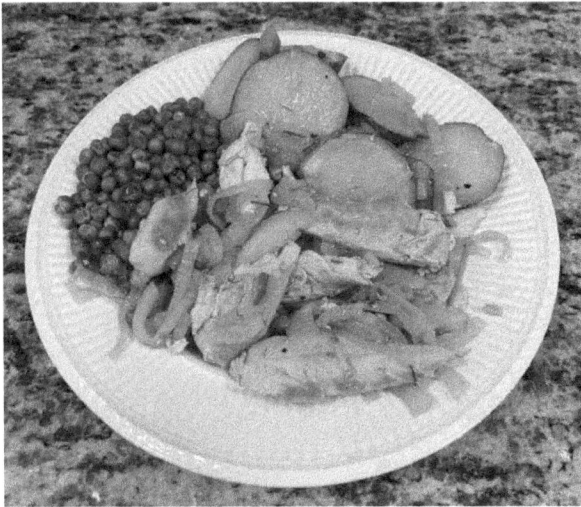

CHICKEN PICATTA WITH ARTICHOKES (6-7 P.M.)

- Coat a large pan with 2-3 tbsp olive oil and place 1 can of artichokes interior side down, brown on medium high heat. Set aside in a bowl for later.

- Add 3-4 cloves of chopped garlic in 2 tbsp olive oil and 1 pound of chick breasts or cutlets, pounded thin. Brown on both sides.

- Whisk together 1 cup sauvignon blanc or other dry white wine, ½ cup of chicken bone broth, 1 tbsp cornstarch, salt and pepper to taste.

- Add back the artichokes and 1 tbsp capers along with the wine mixture. Reduce heat to low and simmer 3-5 minutes or until sauce thickens.

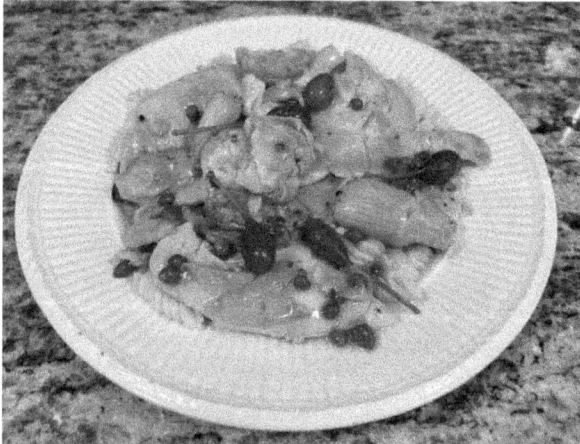

GODFATHER LOUIE'S FISH PASTA (6-7 P.M. BEST DIGESTED ON WEDNESDAY)

- Sauté 1 pound mahi-mahi, or another dense white fish, in 2 tbsp olive oil, remove from pan and clean skin and dark meat if needed.

- Sauté 3-4 cloves of chopped garlic in 2 tbsp olive oil; when they start to brown, add in 1 can of fire-roasted tomatoes, 1 cup of sauvignon blanc or other dry white wine, ¼ cup sliced kalamata olives, salt, and pepper to taste.

- Stir in fish gently and simmer 5 min on low heat. Serve in a bowl over gluten-free pasta.

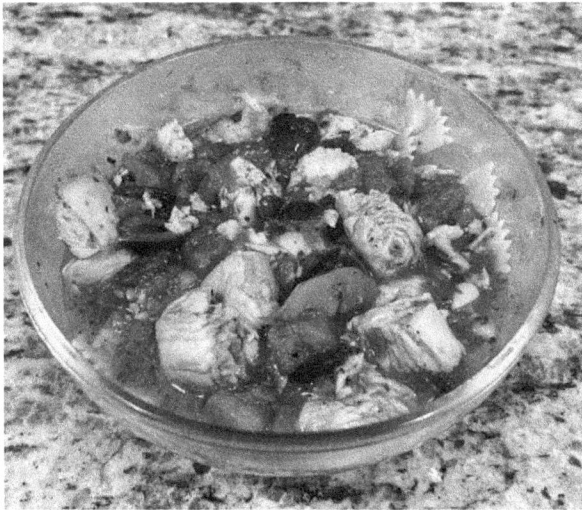

LEMON BASIL CHICKEN (1-3 P.M. IF EATEN ALONE OR 6-7 P.M. IF EATEN WITH PASTA, POTATOES, ETC.)

- Chop 2 cloves garlic and 1 large shallot and put in large pan with 2+ tbsp olive oil, salt, and pepper to taste. I like to use both fresh ground black and white pepper.

- Put 1 pound of chicken breasts or tenders in a Ziploc bag and pound them thin.

- Coat them in the olive oil mixture in the pan by turning them and turn heat onto high (or med high for gas stoves)

- Juice 2 lemons and put juice in a large glass with 1 cup of sauvignon blanc or other white wine and whisk in 1 tbsp cornstarch.

- Flip your chicken. When filets are browned on both sides, add the lemon juice and wine mixture, reduce heat to low, and cover for a few minutes.

- Chop up 1 package of basil (1/4 cup or so) and stir into mixture and remove from heat.

- Garnish with parsley (optional). Eat this solo or with a salad for lunch or serve over gluten-free pasta, or with roasted potatoes and steamed veggies as a side dish if you would like to make it a dinner meal.

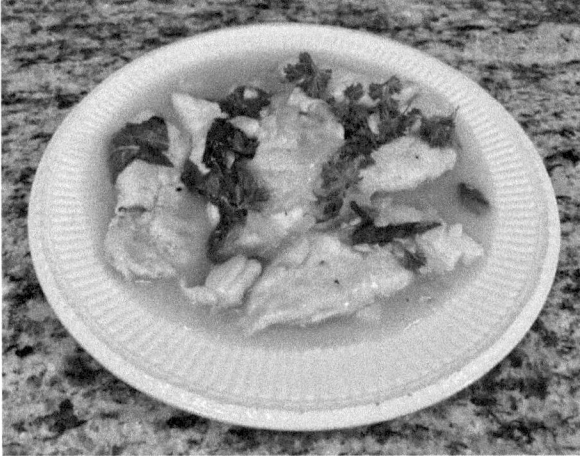

WALNUT CRUSTED SALMON, BROCCOLI, SWEET POTATOES (6-7 P.M.)

- Preheat oven to 425°

- Scrub your sweet potatoes clean and bake until tender, approximately 45 minutes

- Combine salmon topping in a bowl: 1 tsp lemon zest, 2/3 cup chopped walnuts, ½ tsp garlic powder, ½ tsp onion powder, ½ tsp chipotle powder, 1 tbsp Dijon mustard, 2 tbsp maple syrup, 1 tbsp olive oil, salt, and pepper.

- Line a baking sheet with parchment paper and place salmon filets skin side down

- Coat the top of the salmon filets with the topping

- Clean your broccoli and place in a steamer or pot with very little water, don't boil the nutrients out of your veggies

- Put salmon in the oven 6 minutes for every ½-inch of thick thickness–so, a 1-inch-thick filet will be 12 minutes

- Enjoy your potato with grass fed butter and cinnamon

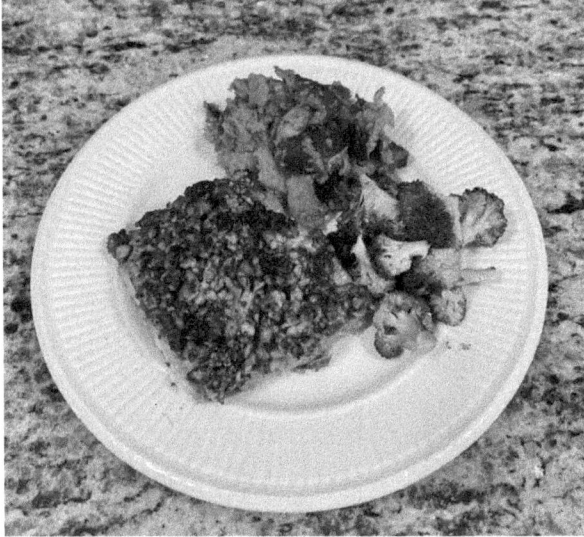

BEEF/BUFFALO PHO (1-3 P.M.)

- Sauté in a large pot

- 1 tbsp fennel seeds

- 1 tbsp coriander seeds

- 2 tbsp coconut oil

- 2 garlic cloves1

- 1 onion

- 1 lb thinly sliced beef or buffalo sirloin

- Add to pot and bring to a boil, then down to simmer for 10 minutes

- 4 cups beef bone broth

- ½ tsp cinnamon

- 1 tsp cloves

- 1 tsp dreid ginger or fresh grated ginger root

- 2 tbsp Tamari

- Turn off heat and stir in 1 package of rice noodles

About the Author

My journey into health and wellness started right out of college. I contracted a urinary tract infection while on vacation and did not go to a doctor for antibiotics. I opted for the Walmart special–Azo Cranberry pills. It spread to my kidneys, and I was forced to go to urgent care where I was given 10 days of Cipro. By the time I was on the 10th day, I had thrush (a yeast infection in the mouth) and new onset digestive problems that persisted for at least a year before I figured out what was going on and was able to regain control of my digestive system. It seemed like I was allergic to everything. I thought I had Crohn's disease. Eventually, I figured out that I had systemic candida overgrowth and with that knowledge, I was able to eliminate my trigger foods, but I still had to take copious amounts of digestive enzymes and probiotics to keep my GI symptoms at bay. This is how I became obsessed with supplements and wellness.

In my late twenties, I decided that being a stressed-out realtor was not what I wanted to do with the rest of my life. I began working in massage as I started the 7-year journey to achieve my Doctorate of Physical Therapy. As I worked on my clients, I had plenty of time to mentor them in the areas of nutrition, supplements, fitness, and overall wellness. I had no idea that health coaching was a "thing." I was just doing it naturally because I wanted to help people.

After earning my Doctor of Physical Therapy, from Florida International University, I began my career at Mount Sinai Hospital in Miami Beach. Working in more hospitals over the span of my career, I noticed a startling trend: Patients are frequently sent home from the hospital without knowing the root cause of their illness. They are left feeling frustrated by the myriad of prescription drugs given as a "band-aid" to cover up their symptoms. We have a sick-care system, not a health-care system. But what if this could all be prevented?

Always believing that nutrition was paramount to good health, becoming a Certified Functional Medicine Practitioner® was the catalyst in the development of a concierge health coaching program for my clients. Becoming a Board-Certified Diplomate with the American Board of Clinical Nutrition was the icing on the [gluten-free] cake!

I founded my online telehealth company because I wanted to empower my patients with the knowledge to understand their bodies and teach them how they can strengthen their immunity through functional medicine testing (lab work done at home) and by treating the root cause of their symptoms with good nutrition, detoxing, and/or nutraceuticals (supplements). Learn more at- **DrSarahDoyle.com.**

As my coaching business grew through my referrals from past client successes, I found that my niche was to help women lose weight, feel better, have increased energy and sex drive. These women are part of the UpWoman® Tribe, where they have completed the 90-day challenge, lost 10-15 pounds, and reclaimed their sexy vibrant youth. As my practice gained more traction, I started getting requests from men, so I created a program for all my guys out there. Most recently, I added a mental health program that works exclusively with brain chemistry. Nutrition is at the core of all my programs and all my clients start with a 7-Day Reset.

See my article on Nutritionalperspectives.org "Case Report: Utilization of Urinary Neurotransmitter Metabolite Testing and Natural Supplements in the Management of Disordered Eating."

There are certain supplements that help balance hormones, but the biggest thing people can do is change their diet. Thus, the 7-Day Nutrition Reset" was born. It is my sincere hope that you implement the 7X Method into your daily life and reap the benefits of improved digestion, increased energy, and increased sexual vitality. Studies show that your sexual vitality is a huge predictor of your overall health![90]

References

1. Jou C. The Progressive Era Body Project: Calorie-Counting and "Disciplining the stomach" in 1920s America. *The Journal of the Gilded Age and Progressive Era.*2019;18(4):422-440. doi:10.1017/S1537781418000348

2. www.mcgill.ca/oss/article/nutrition /how-caloric-value-food-determined

3. USDA

4. Brilliant.org; open.edu

5. Merriam-Webster

6. https://energyeducation.ca/encyclopedia/Photon

7. The Circadian Code: Lose Weight, Supercharge Your Energy, and Transform Your Health from Morning to Midnight: Panda PhD, Satchin: 9781635652437

8. Hastings MH, Maywood ES, Brancaccio M. Generation of circadian rhythms in the suprachiasmatic nucleus. Nat Rev Neurosci. 2018 Aug; 19(8):453-469

9. La Fleur SE, Kalsbeek A, Wortel J, Buijs RM. 1999. A suprachiasmatic nucleus generated rhythm in basal glucose concentrations. *J Neuroendocrinol.* 11:643-652

10. Ruiter M, La Fleur SE, van Heijningen C, van der Vliet J, Kalsbeek A, Buijs RM. 2003. The daily rhythm in plasma glucagon concentrations in the rat is modulated by the biological clock and by feeding behavior. *Diabetes* 52:1709–1715

11. Ando H, Yanagihara H, Hayashi Y, Obi Y, Tsuruoka S, Takamura T, Kaneko S, Fujimura A. 2005. Rhythmic messenger ribonucleic acid expression of clock genes and adipocytokines in mouse visceral adipose tissue. *Endocrinology.* 146:5631–5636

12. De Boer SF, Van der Gugten J. 1987. Daily variations in plasma noradrenaline, adrenaline, and corticosterone concentrations in rats. *Physiol Behav.* 40:323–328

13. Ahima RS, Prabakaran D, Flier JS. 1998. Postnatal leptin surge and regulation of circadian rhythm of leptin by feeding. Implications for energy homeostasis and neuroendocrine function. *J Clin Invest.* 101:1020–1027.;

14. Bodosi B, Gardi J, Hajdu I, Szentirmai E, Obal Jr F, Krueger JM. 2004. Rhythms of ghrelin, leptin, and sleep in rats: effects of the normal diurnal cycle, restricted feeding, and sleep deprivation. *Am J Physiol Regul Integr Comp Physiol.* 287:R1071–R1079.

15. Froy O. 2007. The relationship between nutrition and circadian rhythms in mammals. *Front Neuroendocrinol.*

28:61–71.; Green CB, Takahashi JS, Bass J. 2008. The meter of metabolism. *Cell.* 134:728–742

16. Hirota T, Fukada Y. 2004. Resetting mechanism of central and peripheral circadian clocks in mammals. *Zoolog Sci.* 21:359–368.; Kohsaka A, Bass J. 2007. A sense of time: how molecular clocks organize metabolism. *Trends Endocrinol Metab*18:4–11

17. Voigt R, Summa K, Forsyth C, et al.: The Circadian Clock Mutation Promotes Intestinal Dysbiosis. *Alcoholism: Clinical and Experimental Research 40 (2), 335-347, 2016*

18. Reddy S, Reddy V, Sharma S. Physiology, Circadian Rhythm. [Updated 2021 May 9]. In:StatPearls [Internet]. Treasure Island (FL): StatPearls Publishing; 2021 Jan.

19. Reddy S, Reddy V, Sharma S. Physiology, Circadian Rhythm. [Updated 2021 May 9]. In:StatPearls [Internet]. Treasure Island (FL): StatPearls Publishing; 2021 Jan-

20. The Circadian Code: Lose Weight, Supercharge Your Energy, and Transform Your Health from Morning to Midnight: Panda PhD, Satchin: 9781635652437

21. Segers A, Depoortere I. Circadian Clocks in the Digestive System. *Nature Reviews.*18(239-252). April 2021. doi: 10.1038/s41575-020-00401-5.

22. Circadian clock, Satchin Panda; Brisson, J. Can Poor Digestion Cause Panic Disorder? Part 1: CCK. Digestive Health, Hormones/Neurotransmitters. 2015 Nov 5.

23. University of California–Irvine. "Circadian Clocks: Body parts respond to day and night independently from our brain, studies show." ScienceDaily, 30 May 2019. <www.sciencedaily.com/releases/2019/05/190530141443.htm>

24. Stangherlin, A, Watson JL, Wong, DCS, et al. Compensatory ion transpoprt buffers daily protein rhythms to regulate osmotic balance and cellular physiology. Nat Commun 12, 6035 (2021). https://doi.org/10.1038/s41467-021-25942-4

25. Delisle, B.P., Stumpf, J.L., Wayland, J.L., Johnson, S.R., Ono, M., Hall, D., Burgess, D.E. and Schroder, E.A., 2021. Current Opinion in Pharmacology: Circadian Clocks Regulate Cardiac Arrhythmia Susceptibility, Repolarization, and Ion Channels. *Current opinion in pharmacology*, *57*, p.13

26. Maiese, K., 2020. Cognitive impairment with diabetes mellitus and metabolic disease: innovative insights with the mechanistic target of rapamycin and circadian clock gene pathways. *Expert review of clinical pharmacology*, *13*(1), pp.23-34.

27. West AC, Smith L, Ray DW, et al. Misalignment with the external light environment drives metabolic and cardi-

ac dysfunction. *Nat Commun.* 8, 417 (2017) doi: 10.1038/
s41467-017-00462-2.

28. Eckel-Mahan K, Patel VR, et al. Reprogramming of the Circadian Clock by Nutritional Challenge. *J Cell.* 155(7)1464-1478. Dec 19, 2013. doi: 10.1016/j.cell.2013.11.034

29. Del Campo, J.A., Gallego-Durán, R., Gallego, P. and Grande, L., 2018. Genetic and epigenetic regulation in nonalcoholic fatty liver disease (NAFLD). *International journal of molecular sciences*, 19(3), p.911.

30. Shi, D., Chen, J., Wang, J., Yao, J., Huang, Y., Zhang, G. and Bao, Z., 2019. Circadian clock genes in the metabolism of non-alcoholic fatty liver disease. *Frontiers in physiology*, 10, p.423.

31. Del Campo, J.A., Gallego-Durán, R., Gallego, P. and Grande, L., 2018. Genetic and epigenetic regulation in nonalcoholic fatty liver disease (NAFLD). *International journal of molecular sciences*, 19(3), p.911.

32. Mao Y, Schnytzer Y, Busija L, Churilov L, Davis S, Yan B. "MOONSTROKE": Lunar patterns of stroke occurrence combined with circadian and seasonal rhythmicity–A hospital-based study. *Chronobiology International 32 (7), 881-888, 2015.*

33. Fasano A. All disease begins in the (leaky) gut: role of zonulin-mediated gut permeability in the pathogenesis

of some chronic inflammatory diseases. *F1000Res. 2020 Jan 31;9:F1000 Faculty Rev-69.* doi: 10.12688/f1000research.20510.1 PMID: 32051759; PMCID: PMC6996528

34. Kaczmarek J, Musaad S, Holscher H: Time of day and eating behaviors are associated with the composition and function of the human gastrointestinal microbiota. *The American Journal of Clinical Nutrition* 106 (5), 1220-1231, 2017

35. Bechtold, DA. Energy-responsive timekeeping. *J Genet.* 87, 447-458(2008). doi: 10.1007/s12041-008-0067-6

36. Hernández-Mesa, M., Ropartz, D., García-Campaña, A.M., Rogniaux, H., Dervilly-Pinel, G. and Le Bizec, B., 2019. Ion mobility spectrometry in food analysis: Principles, current applications and future trends. *Molecules, 24*(15), p.2706.

37. https://www.xrite.com/blog/what-does-a-spectrophotometer-measure

38. Hernández-Mesa, M., Ropartz, D., García-Campaña, A.M., Rogniaux, H., Dervilly-Pinel, G. and Le Bizec, B., 2019. Ion mobility spectrometry in food analysis: Principles, current applications and future trends. *Molecules, 24*(15), p.2706

39. Rinawati, M., Sari, L.A. and Pursetyo, K.T., 2020, February. Chlorophyll and carotenoids analysis spectrophotometer using Method on microalgae. In *IOP Conference Se-*

ries: Earth and Environmental Science (Vol. 441, No. 1, p. 012056). IOP Publishing

40. Deidda, R., Sacre, P.Y., Clavaud, M., Coïc, L., Avohou, H., Hubert, P. and Ziemons, E., 2019. Vibrational spectroscopy in analysis of pharmaceuticals: Critical review of innovative portable and handheld NIR and Raman spectrophotometers. *TrAC Trends in Analytical Chemistry*, *114*, pp.251-259

41. Muñiz, R., Cuevas-Valdés, M. and de la Roza-Delgado, B., 2020. Milk quality control requirement evaluation using a handheld near infrared reflectance spectrophotometer and a bespoke mobile application. *Journal of Food Composition and Analysis*, *86*, p.103388.

42. Reddy AB, Karp NA, Maywood ES, et al. Circadian Orchestration of the Hepatic Proteome. *Current Biology.* 16 (11) 1107-1115. June 6, 2006. Doi: 10.1016/j.cub.2006.04.026.

43. Takayasu L, Suda W, Takanashi K, et al.: Circadian oscillations of microbial and functional composition in the human salivary microbiome. *DNA Research* 23 (3), 261-270, 2017

44. Hyman M.: Systems biology, toxins, obesity, and functional medicine. *Altern Ther Health Med* 13 (2), S134-139, 2007

45. D'Adamo D, Whitney C. Eat Right 4 You Blood Type. 2008

46. Ribas-Latre, a, Eckel-Mahan K. Interdependence of nutrient metabolism and the circadian clock system: Importance for metabolic health. *Mol Metab* 5,133-152(2016). doi: 10.1016. j.molmet.2015.12.006

47. Tsoukalas D, Fragkiadaki P, Docea AO, Alegakis AK, Sarandi E, Thanasoula M, Spandidos DA, Tsatsakis A, Razgonova MP, Calina D. Discovery of potent telomerase activators: Unfolding new therapeutic and anti-aging perspectives. Mol Med Rep. 2019 Oct; 20(4):3701-3708. doi: 10.3892/mmr2019.10614. PMID: 31485647; PMCID: PMC6755196

48. www.genome.gov

49. Uchiumi F, Arakawa J, Takihara Y. (2016) The effect of trans-resveratrol on the expression of the human DNA-repair associated genes. Integr Mol Med 3: doi:10.15761/ IMM.1000246

50. Dun A, Zhao X, Jin X, Wei T, Gao X, Wang y, Hou H. Association Between Night-Shift Work and Cancer Risk: Updated Systematic Review and Meta-Analysis. *Front Oncol. 2020 Jun 23;10:1006. doi: 10.3389/fonc.2020.01006. Erratum in : Front Oncol.* 2020 Sep 03;10:1580. PMID: 32656086; PMCID: PMC7324664

51. Ribas-Latre, a, Eckel-Mahan K. Interdependence of nutrient metabolism and the circadian clock system: Impor-

tance for metabolic health. *Mol Metab* 5,133-152(2016). doi: 10.1016. j.molmet.2015.12.006

52. Russell W, Harrison RF, Smith N, Darzy K, Shalet S, Weetman AP, Ross RJ. Free Triiodothyronine Has a Distinct Circadian Rhythm That Is Delayed but Parallels Thyrotropin Levels, *The Journal of Clinical Endocrinology & Metabolism*, Volume 93, Issue 6, 1 June 2008, Pages 2300–2306, doi:10.1210/jc.2007-2674

53. Mehrandish R, Rahimian A, Shahriary A. Heavy metals detoxification: A review of herbal compounds for chelation therapy in heavy metals toxicity. *Journal of Herbmed Pharmacology* 8 (2), 69-77, 2019

54. Segovia-Mendoza M, Nava-Castro KE, Palacios-Arreola MI, Garay-Canales C, Morales-Montor J.: How microplastic components influence the immune system and impact on children health: Focus on Cancer. Birth Defects Res. 2020 Oct;112(17):1341-1361. doi: 10.1002/bdr2.1779. Epub 2020 Aug 6. PMID: 32767490

55. Hwang S, Lim J, Choi Y, J AH. Bisphenol A exposure and type 2 diabetes mellitus risk: a Meta Analysis. *BMC Endocrin Discord.* 2018;18:81. doi:10.1186/s12902-018-0310-y. PMID: 3040086

56. Noonan SC. Oxalate content of foods and its effect on humans. *Asia Pacific journal of clinical nutrition* 8 (1), 64-74, 1999

57. D'Adamo D, Whitney C. Eat Right 4 You Blood Type. 2008

58. Shamsi et al., Metabolic consequences of timed feeding in mice. 2014. *Phys Beh*.128:188-201. doi: 10.1016/j.physbeh.2014.02.021

59. Crosby P, Hamnet R, Putker M, et al; Insulin/IGF-1 drives PERIOD Synthesis to Entrain Circadian Rhythms with Feeding Time. Cell. 2019. 177:896-909. doi: 10.1016/j.cell.2019.02.017

60. Benincasa, P., Falcinelli, B., Lutts, S., Stagnari, F. and Galieni, A., 2019. Sprouted grains: A comprehensive review. *Nutrients*, *11*(2), p.421.

61. Shahidi F et al.:Omega-3 Polyunsaturated Fatty Acids and Their Health Benefits. *Annu Rev Food Sci Technol. 2018*

62. Djurković-Djaković, O., Bobić, B., Nikolić, A., Klun, I. and Dupouy-Camet, J., 2013. Pork as a source of human parasitic infection. *Clinical Microbiology and Infection*, *19*(7), pp.586-594.

63. Schibler et al., Clock Talk: between Central and Peripheral Circadian Oscillators in Mammals. *Cold Spring*

Harb Symp Quant Biol. 2015. 80:223-232. doi: 10.1101/ sqb.2015.80.027490

64. Crosby P, Hamnet R, Putker M, et al; Insulin/IGF-1 drives PERIOD Synthesis to Entrain Circadian Rhythms with Feeding Time. Cell. 2019. 177:896-909. doi: 10.1016/j. cell.2019.02.017

65. Yurtsever T, Schilling TM, Kolsch M, Turner JD, Meyer J, Schachinger H, Schobe AB. 2016.The acute and tempo-rary modulation of PERIOD genesby hydrocortisone in healthy subjects. *Chronobiol Int.* 33:1222-1234;

66. So, A.Y.-L., Bernal, T.U., Pillsbury, M.L., Yamamoto, K.R., and Feldman, B.J. (2009). Glucocorticoid regulation of the cir-cadian clock modulates glucose homeostasis. *Proc. Natl. Acad. Sci. USA* 106, 17582–17587

67. Liu, Lei, et al. "Effect of melatonin on monochromatic light-induced changes in clock gene circadian expression in the chick liver." *Journal of Photochemistry and Photobiol-ogy B: Biology* 197 (2019): 111537. https://doi.org/10.1016/j. jphotobiol.2019.111537

68. Americanredcross.org

69. Leone V, Gibbons S, Martinez K, et al.: Effects of diurnal variation of gut microbes and high-fat feeding on host circadian clock function and metabolism. *Cell host & mi-crobe* 17 (5), 681-689, 2015.

70. Layden B et al.: Short chain fatty acids and their receptors: new metabolic targets. *Transl Res.* 2013 Oct; 162 (4): 269

71. Reddy AB, Karp NA, Maywood ES, et al. Circadian Orchestration of the Hepatic Proteome. *Current Biology.* 16 (11) 1107-1115. June 6, 2006. Doi: 10.1016/j.cub.2006.04.026.

72. Sofer S, Eliraz A, Kaplan S, Voet H, Fink G, Kima T, Madar Z. Greater weight loss and hormonal changes after 6 months diet with carbohydrates eaten mostly at dinner. *Obesity (Silver Spring)*2011;19(10):2006-14

73. D'Adamo D, Whitney C. Eat Right 4 You Blood Type. 2008

74. cancer.gov

75. Trevisan MTS, Owen RW, Calatayud-Vernich P, Breuer A, Pico Y.: Pesticide analysis in coffee leaves using a quick, easy, cheap, effective, rugged and safe approach and liquid chromatography tandem mass spectrometry: Optimization of clean-up step. *Journal of Chromatography A* 1512, 98-106, 2017

76. Utembe W, Kamng'ona AW.: Gut microbiota-mediated pesticide toxicity in humans: methodological issues and challenges in risk assessment of pesticides. *Chemosphere,* 129817, 2021

77. Trevisan MTS, Owen RW, Calatayud-Vernich P, Breuer A, Pico Y.: Pesticide analysis in coffee leaves using a quick,

easy, cheap, effective, rugged and safe approach and liquid chromatography tandem mass spectrometry: Optimization of clean-up step. *Journal of Chromatography A* 1512, 98-106, 2017

78. Kim TW, Lee SH, Choi KH, Kim DH, Han TK. Comparison of the effects of acute exercise after overnight fasting and breakfast on energy substrate and hormone levels in obese men. *Journal of physical therapy science* 27 (6), 1929-1932, 2015

79. Fujiwara T, Nakata R. Skipping breakfast is associated with reproductive dysfunction in post-adolescent female college student. *Appetite.* 2010 Dec; 55(3):714-7. doi: 10.1016/jappet.2010.08.005. Epub 2010 Aug 20. PMID: 20728489

80. Ezagouri, S. et al. Physiological and molecular dissection of daily variance in exercise capacity. Cell Metab. 30, 78–91.e74 (2019)

81. Sakurai M et al.: Skipping breakfast and 5-year changes in body mass index and waist circumference in Japanese men and women. *Obes Sci Pract.* 2017 Apr 3;3(2):162-170. doi:10.1002/osp4.106. PMID: 28702211; PMCID: PMC5478803

82. The Circadian Code: Lose Weight, Supercharge Your Energy, and Transform Your Health from Morning to Midnight: Panda PhD, Satchin: 9781635652437

83. D'Adamo D, Whitney C. Eat Right 4 You Blood Type. 2008

84. The Circadian Code: Lose Weight, Supercharge Your Energy, and Transform Your Health from Morning to Midnight: Panda PhD, Satchin: 9781635652437

85. Fasano A. All disease begins in the (leaky) gut: role of zonulin-mediated gut permeability in the pathogenesis of some chronic inflammatory diseases. *F1000Res. 2020 Jan 31;9:F1000 Faculty Rev-69.* doi: 10.12688/f1000research.20510.1 PMID: 32051759; PMCID: PMC6996528

86. De Palma,G, Collins SM, Bercik P, Verdu EF. The microbiota-gut-brain axis in gastrointestinal disorders: stressed bugs, stressed brain or both? *J Physiol.* 2014;592(14):2989-2997. doi:1113/jphysiol.2014.273995)

87. Circadian clock, Satchin Panda; Brisson, J. Can Poor Digestion Cause Panic Disorder? Part 1: CCK. Digestive Health, Hormones/Neurotransmitters. 2015 Nov 5. <www.fixyourgut.com/can-poor-digestion-cause-panic-disorder-part-1-cck/>

88. Fasano A. All disease begins in the (leaky) gut: role of zonulin-mediated gut permeability in the pathogenesis of some chronic inflammatory diseases. *F1000Res. 2020 Jan 31;9:F1000 Faculty Rev-69.* doi: 10.12688/f1000research.20510.1 PMID: 32051759; PMCID: PMC6996528

89. Fasano A. All disease begins in the (leaky) gut: role of zonulin-mediated gut permeability in the pathogenesis of some chronic inflammatory diseases. *F1000Res. 2020 Jan 31;9:F1000 Faculty Rev-69.* doi: 10.12688/f1000research.20510.1 PMID: 32051759; PMCID: PMC6996528

90. Jackson SE, Yang L, Koyanagi A. et. Al. Declines in Sexual Activity and Function Predict Incident Health Problems in Older Adults: Prospective Findings from the English Longitudinal Study of Ageing. *Arch Sex Behav* 49, 929-940 (2020). https://doi.org/10.1007/s10508-019-1443-4bru

www.ingramcontent.com/pod-product-compliance
Lightning Source LLC
Chambersburg PA
CBHW041928260326
41914CB00009B/1220